Quick Look Nursing:

Nutrition

MARIAN L. FARRELL, PhD, APRN-PMH, CRNP
Professor of Nursing
Department of Nursing
University of Scranton
Scranton, PA

JO ANN L. NICOTERI, PhD(C), APRN, BC, CRNP
Family Nurse Practioner
Department of Nursing/Student Health Services
University of Scranton
Scranton, PA

World Headquarters
Jones and Bartlett Publishers
40 Tall Pine Drive
Sudbury, MA 01776
978-443-5000
info@jbpub.com
www.jbpub.com

Jones and Bartlett Publishers Canada
6339 Ormindale Way
Mississauga, Ontario L5V 1J2
CANADA

Jones and Bartlett Publishers
International
Barb House, Barb Mews
London W6 7PA
UK

Jones and Bartlett's books and products are available through most bookstores and online booksellers. To contact Jones and Bartlett Publishers directly, call 800-832-0034, fax 978-443-8000, or visit our website, www.jbpub.com.

Substantial discounts on bulk quantities of Jones and Bartlett's publications are available to corporations, professional associations, and other qualified organizations. For details and specific discount information, contact the special sales department at Jones and Bartlett via the above contact information or send an email to specialsales@jbpub.com.

The authors, editor, and publisher have made every effort to provide accurate information. However, they are not responsible for errors, omissions, or for any outcomes related to the use of the contents of this book and take no responsibility for the use of the products and procedures described. Treatments and side effects described in this book may not be applicable to all people; likewise, some people may require a dose or experience a side effect that is not described herein. Drugs and medical devices are discussed that may have limited availability controlled by the Food and Drug Administration (FDA) for use only in a research study or clinical trial. Research, clinical practice, and government regulations often change the accepted standard in this field. When consideration is being given to use of any drug in the clinical setting, the health care provider or reader is responsible for determining FDA status of the drug, reading the package insert, and reviewing prescribing information for the most up-to-date recommendations on dose, precautions, and contraindications, and determining the appropriate usage for the product. This is especially important in the case of drugs that are new or seldom used.

Library of Congress Cataloging-in-Publication Data
Farrell, Marian L.
   Nutrition / Marian Farrell, Jo Ann Nicoteri. -- 2nd ed.
     p. ; cm. -- (Quick look nursing)
   Includes bibliographical references and index.
   ISBN-13: 978-0-7637-3739-9
   ISBN-10: 0-7637-3739-9
   1. Nutrition. 2. Nursing. 3. Diet therapy.   I. Nicoteri, Jo Ann L.
II. Title. III. Series.
   [DNLM: 1. Nutrition--Nurses' Instruction.   QU 145 F245n 2007]
RT87.N87F37 2007
613.2--dc22
                                              2006010562
6048

Production Credits
Executive Editor: Kevin Sullivan
Associate Editor: Amy Sibley
Production Director: Amy Rose
Associate Production Editor: Kate Hennessy
Senior Marketing and Project Manager: Emily Ekle
Composition: Shawn Girsberger
Manufacturing and Inventory Coordinator: Amy Bacus
Cover Art: Cara Judd
Cover Design: Timothy Dziewit
Printing and Binding: Malloy, Inc.
Cover Printing: Malloy, Inc

Printed in the United States of America
10 09 08 07 06   10 9 8 7 6 5 4 3 2 1

CONTENTS

PREFACE

The 2005 Dietary Guidelines for Americans (DGAs), released on January 12, 2005, provide nine guidelines for good health. The target audience is policymakers, healthcare providers, and nutrition educators, not the general public.

The DGAs are based on the Dietary Guidelines Advisory Committee's (DGAC) detailed, evidenced-based technical report, recommending easily adoptable daily eating patterns for Americans. The DGAC selected from the food intake data the key nutrients and the important health outcomes, while determining the strength of the relationship between nutrient intake and decreased risk of disease. A food guidance pattern was developed that incorporated nutritious foods, yet allowed for "non-nutritious" foods and cultural diversity.

The 2005 DGAs describe a healthy diet as one that

- emphasizes fruits, vegetables, whole grains, and fat-free or low-fat milk and milk products.
- includes lean meats, poultry, fish, beans, eggs, and nuts.
- is low in saturated fats, trans fats, cholesterol, sodium, and added sugars.

The Food Guide Pyramid changed in 2005 as well. The MyPyramid Plan (Steps to a Healthier You) helps individuals to make smart food choices from every food group; find the balance between food and physical activity; and, get the most nutrition out of consumed calories. Individuals can access the *MyPyramid.gov* website for assistance in developing a plan to choose the foods and amounts that are right for each person.

Dietary Reference Intakes (DRIs), introduced in 1997–1998, have replaced the 1989 Recommended Dietary Allowances (RDAs) as the benchmark of nutrition adequacy in the United States. The Standing Committee on the Scientific Evaluation of Dietary Reference Intakes of the Food and Nutrition Board of the Institute of Medicine completed the review of the entire set of nutrients in 2004. That comprehensive review of the role of nutrients and food components consists of at least three reference values: Estimated Average Requirement (EAR), Recommended Dietary Allowance, and Tolerable Upper Level Intake (UL).

The EAR describes the intake level at which the data indicate that the needs for 50% of those of an age- and gender-specific group consuming it would be met. The Recommended Dietary Allowance is the goal of dietary intake sufficient to meet the nutritional requirements for nearly all individuals in the group. The UL is the maximum level of nutrient intake not likely to cause adverse health effects in nearly all of the individuals in the specific designated group.

This book is intended as an educational tool for health care professionals. Nutrition information is presented across the lifespan, with attention to the most recent recommendations and guidelines for each age group as well as ways to enhance nutritional status. The tables within the text reflect the DRIs (2004) released by the National Academy of Sciences.

M.L.F.
J.A.L.N.

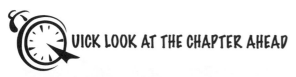

The 2005 USDA Dietary Guidelines:

- Eat more dark green vegetables, orange vegetables, legumes, fruits, whole grains, and low-fat milk and milk products.

- Eat less of refined grains, total fats, added sugars, and calories.

- Eat a variety of nutrient-dense foods and beverages within and among the basic food groups.

- Individuals over age 50 should consume vitamin B_{12} in its crystalline form.

Women who may become pregnant should eat foods high in heme-iron, or iron-rich plant foods, or iron-fortified foods with an enhancer of iron absorption, such as vitamin C, and folic acid from supplements or folate from a varied diet.

Older adults, people with dark skin, and people exposed to insufficient sunlight need to consume extra vitamin D from vitamin D–fortified foods and/or supplements. Recommended total fat intake: 20–30% of total calories for and adult, 30–35% for children ages 2–3, and 25–35% for children and adolescents ages 4–18. Most fats should come from fish, nuts, and vegetable oils. Select and prepare meat, poultry, dry beans, and milk or milk products that are lean, low-fat, or fat-free.

Carbohydrates are found primarily in plant foods and are a source of dietary fiber and energy. Choose fiber-rich whole fruits, vegetables, and whole grains. Whole fruits help meet the fiber requirement. Juice can help meet potassium and calcium requirements. Legumes (e.g., dry beans and peas) should be consumed several times per week. Eat at least half the recommended grain servings as whole grains.

1

Principles of Nutrition: What You Need to Know

TERMS
- ☐ anabolism
- ☐ catabolism
- ☐ marasmus
- ☐ kwashiorkor

1

Nutrition for individuals should come from their dietary intake. The USDA Dietary Guidelines are designed to provide information on selecting nutritious foods, balanced by caloric and energy needs.

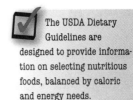

The USDA Dietary Guidelines are designed to provide information on selecting nutritious foods, balanced by caloric and energy needs.

KEY RECOMMENDATIONS OF THE 2005 USDA DIETARY GUIDELINES

- Increase the amount of dark green vegetables, orange vegetables, legumes, fruits, whole grains, and low-fat milk and milk products.
- Decrease the amount of refined grains, total fats, added sugars, and calories.
- Consume a variety of nutrient-dense foods and beverages within and among the basic food groups, while choosing foods that limit the intake of saturated and trans fats, cholesterol, added sugars, salt, and alcohol. (Nutrient-dense foods are those foods that provide large amounts of vitamins and minerals [micronutrients] but few calories; the more an individual consumes of low-density foods the greater likelihood of weight gain.)
- Meet recommended intakes within energy needs by adopting a balanced eating pattern, such as the USDA Food Guide (Figure 1-1) or, in the case of hypertensive individuals, the DASH Eating Plan (Table 1-1).

CONSIDERATIONS FOR SPECIFIC POPULATION GROUPS

- Individuals over age 50 should consume vitamin B_{12} in its crystalline form such as in fortified foods or supplements.
- Women who are in the childbearing age group and may become pregnant are encouraged to eat foods high in heme-iron and/or consume iron-rich plant foods or iron-fortified foods with an enhancer of iron absorption, such as vitamin C–rich foods; they are also advised to consume folic acid daily from fortified foods or supplements, in addition to food forms of folate from a varied diet.
- Older adults, people with dark skin, and people exposed to insufficient ultraviolet-band radiation (i.e., sunlight) need to consume extra vitamin D from vitamin D–fortified foods and/or supplements.

Anatomy of MyPyramid

One size doesn't fit all

USDA's new MyPyramid symbolizes a personalized approach to healthy eating and physical activity. The symbol has been designed to be simple. It has been developed to remind consumers to make healthy food choices and to be active every day. The different parts of the symbol are described below.

Activity

Activity is represented by the steps and the person climbing them, as a reminder of the importance of daily physical activity.

Moderation

Moderation is represented by the narrowing of each food group from bottom to top. The wider base stands for foods with little or no solid fats or added sugars. These should be selected more often. The narrower top area stands for foods containing more added sugars and solid fats. The more active you are, the more of these foods can fit into your diet.

Personalization

Personalization is shown by the person on the steps, the slogan, and the URL. Find the kinds and amounts of food to eat each day at MyPyramid.gov.

Proportionality

Proportionality is shown by the different widths of the food group bands. The widths suggest how much food a person should choose from each group. The widths are just a general guide, not exact proportions. Check the Web site for how much is right for you.

Variety

Variety is symbolized by the 6 color bands representing the 5 food groups of the Pyramid and oils. This illustrates that foods from all groups are needed each day for good health.

Gradual improvement

Gradual improvement is encouraged by the slogan. It suggests that individuals can benefit from taking small steps to improve their diet and lifestyle each day.

MyPyramid.gov
STEPS TO A HEALTHIER YOU

| GRAINS | VEGETABLES | FRUITS | OILS | MILK | MEAT & BEANS |

USDA U.S. Department of Agriculture
Center for Nutrition Policy
and Promotion
April 2005 CNPP-16

USDA is an equal opportunity provider and employer

Figure 1-1 Anatomy of MyPyramid

The DASH eating plan shown below is based on 2,000 calories a day. The number of daily servings in a food group may vary from those listed, depending on your caloric needs. Use this chart to help you plan your menus or take it with you when you go to the store.

Food Group	Daily Servings (EXCEPT AS NOTED)	Serving Sizes	Examples and Notes	Significance of Each Food Group to the DASH Eating Plan
Grains and grain products	7–8	1 slice bread 1 oz dry cereal* $1/2$ cup cooked rice, pasta, or cereal	Whole wheat bread, English muffin, pita bread, bagel, cereals, grits, oatmeal, crackers, unsalted pretzels and popcorn	Major sources of energy and fiber
Vegetables	4–5	1 cup raw leafy vegetable $1/2$ cup cooked vegetable 6 oz vegetable juice	Tomatoes, potatoes, carrots, green peas, squash, broccoli, turnip greens, collards, kale, spinach, artichokes, green beans, lima beans, sweet potatoes	Rich sources of potassium, magnesium, and fiber
Fruits	4–5	6 oz fruit juice 1 medium fruit $1/4$ cup dried fruit $1/2$ cup fresh, frozen, or canned fruit	Apricots, bananas, dates, grapes, oranges, orange juice, grapefruit, grapefruit juice, mangoes, melons, peaches, pineapples, prunes, raisins, strawberries, tangerines	Important sources of potassium, magnesium, and fiber
Lowfat or fat free dairy foods	2–3	8 oz milk 1 cup yogurt $1 1/2$ oz cheese	Fat free (skim) or lowfat (1%) milk, fat free or lowfat buttermilk, fat free or lowfat regular or frozen yogurt, lowfat and fat free cheese	Major sources of calcium and protein
Meats, poultry, and fish	2 or less	3 oz cooked meats, poultry, or fish	Select only lean; trim away visible fats; broil, roast, or boil, instead of frying; remove skin from poultry	Rich sources of protein and magnesium
Nuts, seeds, and dry beans	4–5 per week	$1/3$ cup or $1 1/2$ oz nuts 2 Tbsp or $1/2$ oz seeds $1/2$ cup cooked dry beans peas	Almonds, filberts, mixed nuts, peanuts, walnuts, sunflower seeds, kidney beans, lentils,	Rich sources of energy, magnesium, potassium, protein, and fiber
Fats and oils†	2–3	1 tsp soft margarine 1 Tbsp lowfat mayonnaise 2 Tbsp light salad dressing 1 tsp vegetable oil	Soft margarine, lowfat mayonnaise, light salad dressing, vegetable oil (such as olive, corn, canola, or safflower)	DASH has 27 percent of calories as fat, including fat in or added to foods
Sweets	5 per week	1 Tbsp sugar 1 Tbsp jelly or jam $1/2$ oz jelly beans 8 oz lemonade	Maple syrup, sugar, jelly, jam, fruit-flavored gelatin, jelly beans, hard candy, fruit punch, sorbet, ices	Sweets should be low in fat

* Equals $1/2$ – $1 1/4$ cups, depending on cereal type. Check the product's Nutrition Facts Label.
† Fat content changes serving counts for fats and oils: For example, 1 Tbsp of regular salad dressing equals 1 serving; 1 Tbsp of a lowfat dressing equals $1/2$ serving; 1 Tbsp of a fat free dressing equals 0 servings.

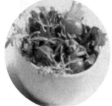

Table 1-1 Following the DASH Eating Plan

It is important for individuals to remember that their dietary intake needs to provide all of the nutrients for growth and health. Since each basic food group is a major contributor to a balanced diet, it is important to include a variety of all of the food groups on a daily basis. Individuals also need to be aware of selecting nutrient-dense foods since they provide a greater amount of vitamins and minerals and relatively fewer calories.

VITAMINS

Vitamins are organic compounds essential for normal functioning and growth and maintenance of the body. Vitamins are not a source of energy. Vitamins are required in very small amounts and serve a number of functions in the body, such as regulating chemical reactions.

Since vitamins are not synthesized in the body, there must be a dietary intake. The Dietary Reference Intakes (DRIs) reflect the requirements necessary to prevent deficiencies, as well as toxicity, from overdoses of vitamins.

A primary deficiency of a vitamin occurs when the vitamin is not consumed in sufficient amounts to meet physiological needs. A secondary deficiency develops when absorption is impaired or excess excretion occurs, limiting bioavailability of the vitamin.

There are two categories of vitamins: water-soluble and fat-soluble. Water-soluble vitamins dissolve or disperse in water. Examples of water-soluble vitamins include vitamin C and vitamin Bs (thiamine, riboflavin, niacin, folate, vitamin B_6, vitamin B_{12}, biotin, and pantothenic acid).

> It is important for individuals to remember that their dietary intake needs to provide all of the nutrients for growth and health. Since each basic food group is a major contributor to a balanced diet, it is important to include a variety of all of the food groups on a daily basis. Individuals also need to be aware of selecting nutrient-dense foods since they provide a greater amount of vitamins and minerals and relatively fewer calories.

> Bioavailability is the rate and extent to which a metabolite enters the general circulation.

> Examples of water-soluble vitamins include vitamin C and vitamin Bs (thiamine, riboflavin, niacin, folate, vitamin B_6, vitamin B_{12}, biotin, and pantothenic acid).

- Water-soluble vitamins are more easily absorbed in the small intestine.
- There is minimal storage of any excess.
- Excesses are generally not toxic and are simply excreted in urine.
- Deficiencies develop quickly when water-soluble vitamins are not consumed daily.
- Damage may result if vitamin levels are chronically high, owing to supplementation.

Fat-soluble vitamins dissolve in fatty tissues or substance. Fat-soluble vitamins include vitamins A, D, E, and K.

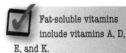
Fat-soluble vitamins include vitamins A, D, E, and K.

- Bile is necessary for the absorption of fat-soluble vitamins from the small intestine.
- Excesses are stored in the liver and spleen and other fatty tissues.
- Overloading of fat-soluble vitamins can be toxic and produce illness.

MINERALS

Minerals serve a variety of functions.

- Minerals provide rigidity and strength to the teeth and skeleton.
- Skeletal mineral components serve as a storage depot for other needs of the body.
- Nerve and muscle functions are influenced by minerals, allowing for proper muscle contraction and release.
- Minerals help maintain the proper acid-base balance of body fluids and are required for blood clotting, tissue repair, and growth.

There are two categories of minerals: major and trace. Major minerals are essential nutrient minerals required daily in amounts of 100 mg or higher. Trace minerals are essential nutrient minerals required daily in amounts less than 100 mg.

Trace minerals serve as cofactors for enzymes, components of hormones, and participants in oxidation-reduction reactions. Trace minerals are essential for growth and for normal functioning of the immune system. It is important to recognize that the classification of major and trace minerals is unrelated to importance.

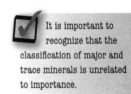
It is important to recognize that the classification of major and trace minerals is unrelated to importance.

Lack of trace minerals may cause delayed sexual maturation, poor growth, faulty immune function, altered hormonal function, and tooth decay. The recommended DRI for vitamins and minerals is listed in Appendix A.

Both plants and animals are sources of minerals. Animal sources tend to be more consistent sources than plant foods, which vary depending upon the plant, soil, and mineral. Another consideration is bioavailability.

Since the gastrointestinal tract absorbs a smaller proportion of minerals than of vitamins, it is important not to megadose certain minerals, such as calcium.

Many minerals tend to have similar chemical properties and will compete for absorption. Dietary fiber will also affect absorption.

PROTEINS

Proteins consist of chains of amino acids. There are nine essential amino acids (essential because they cannot be produced by the body and require food sources). The number of nonessential amino acids totals 11 and they are created by the liver. Proteins help build tissue and fill a variety of physiological roles. Examples include hormones, enzymes, and antibodies. Protein formation is called **anabolism**, and protein breakdown is called **catabolism**.

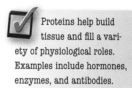
Proteins help build tissue and fill a variety of physiological roles. Examples include hormones, enzymes, and antibodies.

The proteins in foods are categorized by the essential amino acids they contain. Complete proteins contain all nine essential amino acids, while incomplete proteins lack one or more. The proteins in foods are not the same as those used by the body.

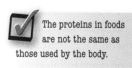
The proteins in foods are not the same as those used by the body.

During digestion, food protein is broken down to amino acids. Once absorbed, the amino acids circulate in the blood to build new proteins. The new proteins perform numerous functions, including growth and maintenance, creation of essential substances, immune system response, fluid regulation, acid-base balance, and transportation of nutrients and other substances in the body.

> Inadequate intake of protein leads to conditions of malnutrition known as **marasmus** and **kwashiorkor**.

The AMDR (Accepted Macronutrient Distribution Range) for protein is 10 to 35% of calories.

FATS

Fats include a broad range of organic molecules. The main classes of fats found in foods and in the body are triglycerides, phospholipids, and sterols. The largest category, triglycerides, are found in foods and in adipose tissue in the body.

Phospholipids are found in both plant and animals and play a crucial role in cell membranes and in blood and body fluid, where they help keep fats suspended in fluid and serve as emulsifiers.

Sterols are a small percentage of dietary lipids, and include cholesterol, which comes from food and is also made by the body. Cholesterol is an important component of cell membranes and an important precursor in the synthesis of sex hormones, vitamin D, and bile acids.

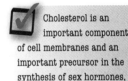

Cholesterol is an important component of cell membranes and an important precursor in the synthesis of sex hormones, vitamin D, and bile acids.

Lipids share similar functional properties, solubility, and transport mechanisms, although the composition and structure of individual molecules varies. Fatty acids are components of both triglycerides and phospholipids, and are often attached to cholesterol.

- Fatty acids will determine the characteristics of a fat, whether it is a solid or a liquid.
- A free fatty acid is one that is not joined to another compound.
- Fatty acids differ in chain length—the shorter the chain length the more liquid, the lower the melting point, the more water soluble, and the higher the absorption.
- A saturated fatty acid is viewed as fully loaded with hydrogen if all the carbon in the chain is joined with single bonds and the remaining bonds are filled with hydrogen.
- An unsaturated fatty acid is one that has fewer hydrogen bonds, so the chain is not saturated.

The functions of lipids fall into two categories: food-value functions and physiological functions. Lipids that have food-value functions include the fat that is the densest form of stored energy in both food and the body.

Lipids that have physiological functions include fats that are stored and provide a backup energy supply, cushion body organs, and serve to regulate body temperature.

Digestion of lipids occurs mainly in the small intestine. The absorption rate depends on the transportation of lipids through the lymph and blood circulatory systems.

Saturated fats tend to remain solid at room temperature. Unsaturated fats tend to remain liquid at room temperature.

Fats are important because they supply energy and essential fatty acids. Fats also assist in the absorption of fat-soluble vitamins A, D, E, and K and carotenoids.

> Fats are important because they supply energy and essential fatty acids. Fats also assist in the absorption of fat-soluble vitamins A, D, E, and K and carotenoids.

Individuals who consume a high intake (greater than 35% of calories) of saturated fats, trans fats, and cholesterol are at increased risk of coronary heart disease.

Key Recommendations

- The recommended total fat intake for an adult is between 20 and 35% of total calories consumed.
- A fat intake of 30 to 35% is recommended for children 2 to 3 years of age.
- For children and adolescents 4 to 18 years of age, 25 to 35% is recommended.
- Adults need to decrease their intake of saturated fat and trans fats and usually their dietary intake of cholesterol.
- Consume less than 10% of total calories from saturated fatty acids and less than 300 mg/day of cholesterol, and keep trans fatty acid consumption as low as possible.
- Keep total fat intake between 20 to 35% of total calories, with most fats coming from sources of polyunsaturated and monounsaturated fatty acids, such as fish, nuts, and vegetable oils.

- Select and prepare meat, poultry, dry beans, and milk or milk products that are lean, low-fat, or fat-free.
- Limit intake of fats and oils high in saturated and/or trans fatty acids.
- Choose products low in fats and oils.

CARBOHYDRATES

Carbohydrates are organic, found primarily in plant foods, and serve as an abundant source of dietary fiber and energy. The two main types of carbohydrates in food are simple carbohydrates (sugars) and complex carbohydrates (starches and fiber). The reported benefits of dietary fiber include decreased constipation and decreased risks of coronary heart disease, gastrointestinal disorders, and type 2 diabetes.

> ✓ The two main types of carbohydrates in food are simple carbohydrates (sugars) and complex carbohydrates (starches and fiber).

Sugars and starches supply the body with energy in the form of glucose.

It is important to choose carbohydrates that provide the appropriate selection of nutrients while not increasing the calories to the point of weight gain.

The AMDR for carbohydrates is 45 to 65% of total calories.

Key Recommendations

- Choose fiber-rich fruits, vegetables, and whole grains.
- Pick whole fruits rather than fruit juice to help meet the fiber requirement.
- Fruit juice can help meet potassium and calcium requirements.
- Select and prepare foods and beverages with little added sugars or caloric sweeteners.
- Consume 14 g of dietary fiber per 1000 cal.
- Legumes (e.g., dry beans and peas) should be consumed several times per week.
- Eat whole grains for at least half the recommended total servings of grain.

SPECIFIC POPULATION GROUPS

Approximately 20% of adults over 65 may be affected by constipation, due to lack of dietary fiber, drug interaction, and decreased hydration.

Children and adolescents tend to take in too much carbohydrate, often associated with too many calories and inadequate dietary fiber. Obesity and dental caries are associated with increased consumption of sweetened dairy foods, beverages, and cereals. Recommendations for this age group include increased consumption of whole fruits, vegetables, and whole-grain products. Sample menus for a 2000-calorie food pattern are available in Appendix B.

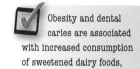

Obesity and dental caries are associated with increased consumption of sweetened dairy foods, beverages, and cereals.

CHAPTER 1 • QUESTIONS

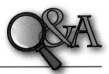

1. What type of deficiency is impaired absorption or excess excretion of a vitamin?
   a. Primary deficiency
   b. Secondary deficiency
   c. Tertiary deficiency
   d. Catenary deficiency

2. Fat-soluble vitamins dissolve in fatty tissues, and include vitamins A, D, E, and what other vitamin?
   a. C
   b. K
   c. B_6
   d. B_{12}

3. To absorb vitamins from the intestine, what substance is required to be present?
   a. Bile
   b. Lipase
   c. Cholesterol
   d. Bilirubin

4. Major minerals (essential nutrient minerals) are required daily in what amounts of milligrams?
   a. 10 mg
   b. 20 mg
   c. 50 mg
   d. 100 mg

5. What is the recommended AMDR of protein for adults as a percentage of total calories?
   a. 5 to 10%
   b. 10 to 15%
   c. 20 to 25%
   d. 10 to 35%

6. There are how many essential amino acids?
    a. 9
    b. 12
    c. 15
    d. 20

7. What is the largest category of fats?
    a. Bile
    b. Steroids
    c. Cholesterol
    d. Triglycerides

8. Where does digestion of lipids mainly occur?
    a. Stomach
    b. Gallbladder
    c. Small intestine
    d. Large intestine

9. What are the fats that remain solid at room temperature called?
    a. Saturated
    b. Unsaturated
    c. Conjugated
    d. Unconjugated

10. What is the AMDR for carbohydrates?
    a. 10 to 15%
    b. 20 to 25%
    c. 30 to 40%
    d. 45 to 65%

CHAPTER 1 • ANSWERS AND RATIONALES

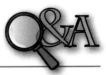

1. **The answer is b.** Secondary deficiency occurs due to impaired absorption or excess excretion, which limits bioavailability of the vitamins. Primary deficiency occurs when the vitamin is not consumed in sufficient amounts.

2. **The answer is b.** Vitamins C, B_6, B_{12} are water-soluble vitamins.

3. **The answer is a.** Bile is an enzyme secreted by the liver and stored in the gallbladder. Lipase is an enzyme that catalyzes the breakdown of lipid. Cholesterol is a lipid that facilitates the absorption and transport of fatty acids. Bilirubin is formed from the breakdown of hemoglobin in red blood cells.

4. **The answer is d.** Trace minerals are required in amounts less than 20 mg.

5. **The answer is d.**

6. **The answer is a.**

7. **The answer is d.**

8. **The answer is c.**

9. **The answer is a.** Unsaturated fats remain liquid at room temperature.

10. **The answer is d.**

Preconceptual counseling helps a woman to make decisions that will improve the outcome of her pregnancy.

Adolescents must meet their own growth needs as well as the requirements of pregnancy. Yet young adolescents (ages 11–15) are likely to eat fast foods and engage in chronic dieting to conceal the pregnancy.

Women age 40+ are more likely to have such pre-existing conditions as hypertension and diabetes, which raise the risk of low birth weight and pre-term delivery. Diabetes mellitus can produce a macrosomic (overly large) baby.

Women who have multiple pregnancies with close spacing have a high risk of delivering low-birth-weight babies, of prematurity, and of having spontaneous abortions.

Obese women (BMI > 30 kg/m²) should gain only ~7 kg. Underweight women (BMI < 19.8 kg/m²) may gain up to 18 kg. Average-weight women may gain 1.4–2.3 kg/month during the first trimester and 0.5–0.9 kg/week during the rest of the pregnancy.

Many women experience nausea and vomiting during pregnancy, especially during the first trimester, alleviated by eating small amounts of food every 3 to 4 hours and avoiding eating and drinking fluids at the same time.

During pregnancy, women should eat a well-balanced diet and engage in sufficient exercise. Inappropriate maternal weight gain and pica can place the newborn at greater risk for infection, illness, disabilities, and even death.

2

Pregnancy

TERMS
- [ ] pica
- [ ] caffeine
- [ ] maternal parity

Caffeine consumption during pregnancy decreases the blood flow through the placenta, increases the risk of spontaneous abortion during the first trimester, and may lead to caffeine withdrawal symptoms in the newborn.

Several factors affect the outcome of pregnancy. One of the most important is preconceptual counseling, which helps a woman to make decisions that will improve the outcome of her pregnancy. Planning for positive pregnancy outcomes needs to occur across all socioeconomic and educational levels.

Factors such as age, parity, maternal weight prior to pregnancy, cultural and religious beliefs, economic status, education, occupation, cigarette smoking, drinking alcohol, and patterns of eating all have an impact on the outcome of a pregnancy.

Factors such as age, parity, maternal weight prior to pregnancy, cultural and religious beliefs, economic status, education, occupation, cigarette smoking, drinking alcohol, and patterns of eating all have an impact on the outcome of a pregnancy.

Young pregnant adolescents (11–15 years of age) are likely to experience nutritional deficits. Adolescents must meet their own growth needs as well as the requirements of pregnancy. They are also likely to eat fast foods and engage in chronic dieting, in an attempt to conceal the pregnancy.

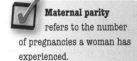

Maternal parity refers to the number of pregnancies a woman has experienced.

Women age 40 and over are considered to be at high risk because they are more likely to have preexisting conditions, such as hypertension and diabetes, that can negatively affect pregnancy. Hypertension and diabetes place a pregnant woman at significant risk for low birth weight and preterm delivery. In some cases women who have diabetes mellitus will have a large baby, which is referred to as macrosomia.

Maternal parity refers to the number of pregnancies a woman has experienced. In addition to her parity, it is important to know the spacing of a woman's pregnancies. Women who have multiple pregnancies with close spacing are at risk of bearing low-birth-weight or premature babies and experiencing spontaneous abortions.

A woman's prepregnancy BMI (body mass index) is used as a basis for planning weight management. For women who are obese (BMI > 30 kg/m²), the recommended goal should be a small weight gain of ~7 kg. If women are underweight (BMI < 19.8 kg/m²) more weight gain is allowable (up to 18 kg). For average-weight women, a gain of 1.4 to 2.3 kg/month during the first trimester and 0.5 to 0.9 kg/week during the rest of the pregnancy is recommended.

Cultural and religious beliefs influence how a woman lives each day. Her value belief system affects every aspect of her life, such as what she eats, her wake/sleep pattern, her system of self-care, and her social support system.

Economic status affects a woman's food budget, her housing, and her ability to obtain daily support. Education influences the woman's occupation, finances, level of knowledge, and level of understanding. It also influences the decisions a woman makes regarding her lifestyle and care. Occupation may present worksite conditions that put both the woman and her fetus at risk. In addition, occupation may affect fertility for some women.

FACTORS AFFECTING NUTRITION DURING PREGNANCY

Many women experience nausea and vomiting during pregnancy, especially during the first trimester. The nausea can be the result of an accumulation of gastric acid in the stomach. This can be alleviated by eating small amounts of food every 3 to 4 hours. Some women also benefit from eating dry toast or crackers, especially if they are nauseated when they first wake up in the morning. It is also important to avoid eating and drinking fluids at the same time.

Toward the end of pregnancy, many women will experience a return of nausea, which is often attributed to decreased gastric peristalsis. Again, eating small meals frequently may be helpful.

Women need to have bulk in their diet and to maintain exercise at an appropriate level, which also helps them to be less constipated. Food aversion, heartburn, weight gain, hemorrhoids, lactose intolerance, and

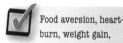 Food aversion, heartburn, weight gain, hemorrhoids, lactose intolerance, and vegetarianism can all have a negative impact on pregnant women and the outcome of the pregnancy.

vegetarianism can all have a negative impact on pregnant women and the outcome of the pregnancy.

During pregnancy, women need to eat a well-balanced diet that has sufficient calories and represents a variety of food groups. They need to be encouraged to maintain a healthy diet and sufficient exercise throughout pregnancy. Inappropriate weight gain can place the newborn at greater risk for infection, illness, disabilities, and even death. Some women experience pica cravings. **Pica** is eating substances like clay that have no nutrient value.

> **Pica** is eating substances like clay that have no nutrient value.

Pica may lessen the nutritional level of the mother and her fetus since the mother may not eat nutritious foods in sufficient quantity, which can lead to poor weight gain, low birth weight, and intrauterine growth retardation. Also, the substance that the woman is eating may have harmful effects on the mother and her fetus.

Women who drink two to three cups of coffee each day have a caffeine intake of about 300mg/day.

Caffeine decreases the absorption of iron, which has a direct impact on mother and fetus. During pregnancy, caffeine decreases blood flow through the placenta and also increases the risk of spontaneous abortion during the first trimester. Caffeine consumption during pregnancy may also lead to caffeine withdrawal symptoms in the newborn.

Four non-nutritive sweeteners (saccharin, aspartame, acesulfame-K, and sucralose) have been approved by the FDA as safe for consumption during pregnancy, but moderation is recommended.

ADVICE FOR NURSES

Point Out Common Behaviors That Affect Pregnancy

- Drinking alcohol
- Taking drugs
- Drinking caffeinated beverages
- Smoking

- Having an eating disorder
- Exercising
- Persistently eating foods with no nutrient value (pica)
- Dieting
- Eating a vegetarian diet
- Taking oral contraceptives

Suggest Ways to Enhance Nutrition

- Increase folic acid intake
- Attend educational classes on nutrition
- Increase the compliance factor
- Participate in preconceptual counseling
- Receive early, routine prenatal care

Questions to Ask the Mother

What have you eaten in the past 24 hours (a 24-hour recall)?

What is your normal weight pattern?

What is your normal pattern of food intake?

What type (if any) of vitamin and mineral supplements do you take?

Do you have any food allergies or intolerance?

Do you have any preexisting medical conditions (anemia, diabetes mellitus, hypertension, cardiac, renal)?

Do you have an eating disorder (anorexia, bulimia, bingeing)?

What are the cultural influences on your dietary intake?

CHAPTER 2 · QUESTIONS

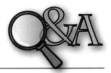

1. What is the expected weight gain in pounds for a woman during pregnancy?
   a. 10–15 lbs
   b. 15–20 lbs
   c. 20–25 lbs
   d. 25–30 lbs

2. Nausea experienced by pregnant women is due to an accumulation of what substance in the stomach?
   a. Trypsin
   b. Amylase
   c. Gastric acid
   d. Lipase

3. Nausea in pregnant women can be lessened if they eat small meals every _____ hours each day:
   a. 1–2
   b. 2–3
   c. 3–4
   d. 4–5

4. During pregnancy, what is the term for women eating foods that have no nutrient value?
   a. Pica
   b. Mellitus
   c. Anorexia
   d. Bulimia

5. A pregnant woman should gain how many kilograms per week during the second and third trimesters?
   a. 0.5 to 0.9 Kg
   b. 1.0 to 2.2 Kg
   c. 2.4 to 3.0 Kg
   d. 3.2 to 4.0 Kg

6. Toward the end of pregnancy many women will experience a return of nausea which is often attributed to:
    a. Tight clothing
    b. Increased glucose in diet
    c. Fetus has increased scalp and body hair
    d. Decreased gastric peristalsis

7. Pregnant women can decrease the risk of constipation by maintaining exercise and:
    a. Using stool softeners
    b. Increasing bulk in their diet
    c. Enemas
    d. Decreasing their fluid intake

8. The use of this substance by pregnant women decreases the absorption of iron, reduces the blood flow to the placenta, and increases the risk of spontaneous abortion:
    a. Caffeine
    b. Aspartame
    c. Nicotene
    d. MSG

9. The total folic acid requirements during pregnancy is:
    a. 200 mg/day
    b. 400 mg/day
    c. 600 mg/day
    d. 800 mg/day

CHAPTER 2 · ANSWERS AND RATIONALES

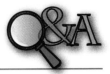

1. The answer is d.

2. The answer is c. Trypsin is an enzyme that catalyzes in the small intestine. Amylase is an enzyme that catalyzes the hydrolysis of starch into smaller carbohydrate molecules. Lipase is an enzyme that catalyzes the breakdown of lipids.

3. The answer is c.

4. The answer is a. Mellitus is referring to diabetes mellitus, a disturbance in glucose metabolism. Anorexia refers to restricting dietary intake. Bulimia refers to purging behaviors.

5. The answer is a.

6. The answer is d.

7. The answer is b.

8. The answer is a.

9. The answer is c.

Women need to increase their calories by 300 per day during the second and third trimester of pregnancy. The expected weight gain is an average of 25 to 30 pounds.

Pregnancy is not a time for dieting; weight loss can result in maternal ketosis and low birth weight.

Obese women have an increased incidence of diabetes mellitus, leading to macrosomic babies, and they are at increased risk for high blood pressure and blood lipids.

Carbohydrates provide protective functions, fiber, and energy. The recommended carbohydrate intake is 175 g/day. If total calorie intake is not adequate, protein breaks down, which leads to ketosis.

Protein provides amino acids for fetal development, blood volume expansion, and growth of maternal tissues such as the breasts and the uterus, and contributes to overall energy metabolism. The recommended protein intake is 71 g/day. Good sources of protein are meat, fish, poultry, eggs, dairy products (milk, yogurt, cheese, and custards), soy milk, tofu, or soybean products.

Dietary cholesterol, trans fatty acids, and saturated fatty acids need to be kept as low as possible, while consuming a nutritionally adequate diet during pregnancy. Added sugars should not be more than 25% of the total energy.

3

Nutrition Facts Related to Pregnancy: Carbohydrates, Protein, and Fats

TERMS
- [ ] **ketosis**
- [ ] **amino acids**

Women need to increase their calories by 300 calories per day during the second and third trimesters. The expected weight gain is an average of 25 to 30 lb. An optimal weight gain during pregnancy depends upon a woman's weight for height (BMI).

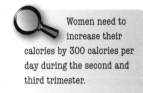

Women need to increase their calories by 300 calories per day during the second and third trimester.

Pregnancy is not a time for dieting, since decreased food intake can result in maternal ketosis. Women who are below their recommended weight are likely to deliver a low-birth-weight newborn.

During the second trimester, most of the weight gain reflects an increase in blood volume, enlargement of breasts, uterus, tissue, and fluid.

Obese women have an increased incidence of diabetes mellitus and macrosomic (large) babies. Women who are above the recommended weight are also at increased risk for high blood pressure and increased blood lipids.

CARBOHYDRATES

The recommended carbohydrate intake during pregnancy is 175 g/day. See Appendix A for dietary calculations and additional macronutrients. Carbohydrates provide protective functions, fiber, and energy. If total calorie intake is not adequate, the body uses protein for energy, and thus protein is not available for body building. When protein breaks down, this leads to ketosis. **Ketosis** (especially in diabetic women) is due to glycosuria, reduced alkaline reserves, and lipidemia. Women need to be encouraged to maintain a healthy diet through the use of dairy products, fruits, vegetables, and whole-grain cereals and bread.

Ketosis (especially in diabetic women) is due to glycosuria, reduced alkaline reserves, and lipidemia.

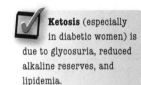

Women need to be encouraged to maintain a healthy diet through the use of dairy products, fruits, vegetables, and whole-grain cereals and bread.

PROTEIN

The recommended protein intake during pregnancy is 71 g/day. Protein is needed in increased amounts to provide amino acids for fetal development, blood volume expansion, and growth of maternal tissues, such as the breasts and the uterus. Also, protein contributes to overall energy metabolism. The quality of proteins is important and is determined by the complex of **amino acids** necessary to sustain growth. Good sources of protein are meat, fish, poultry, eggs, and dairy products (milk, yogurt, cheese, and custards). If the pregnant woman is lactose intolerant, allergic to dairy products, or vegetarian, she may use soy milk, tofu, or soybean products.

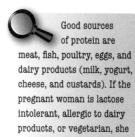

Good sources of protein are meat, fish, poultry, eggs, and dairy products (milk, yogurt, cheese, and custards). If the pregnant woman is lactose intolerant, allergic to dairy products, or vegetarian, she may use soy milk, tofu, or soybean products.

FATS

Fats provide a valuable source of energy. Since fats are more completely absorbed during pregnancy, pregnant women experience increases in serum lipids, lipoprotein, and cholesterol, and decreased elimination of fat through the bowel. Dietary cholesterol, trans fatty acids, and saturated fatty acids need to be kept as low as possible, while consuming a nutritionally adequate diet during pregnancy. Added sugars should not be more than 25% of the total.

Questions to Ask the Mother

What significance do you place on food?
What has been the frequency of your prenatal visits?
What is your daily food intake?
Have you experienced any weight gain or loss?
What is your caffeine consumption?
Have you noticed the presence of swelling on your face, hands, or feet; headaches; or spots before your eyes?
Have there been changes in your blood pressure?
How does your culture, ethnicity, and religion affect your food intake?
What is your aspartame consumption (e.g., NutraSweet and Equal)?

CHAPTER 3 • QUESTIONS

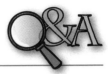

1. During pregnancy, what is the recommended intake of carbohydrates?
   a. 100 g
   b. 135 g
   c. 175 g
   d. 200 g

2. During pregnancy, what should the DRI of protein be?
   a. 51 g
   b. 61 g
   c. 71 g
   d. 81 g

3. During pregnancy, women need to increase their total number of calories by how much?
   a. 200 calories
   b. 300 calories
   c. 400 calories
   d. 500 calories

4. What chronic illness, in addition to hypertension, is likely to cause high-risk pregnancies for women 40 years and older?
   a. Heart disease
   b. Renal disease
   c. System lupus
   d. Diabetes mellitus

5. When protein breaks down, this leads to:
   a. Ketosis
   b. Proteinuria
   c. Fatty acids
   d. Glucose

6. Because fats are more completely absorbed during pregnancy, women are more likely to experience which of the following disorders?
   a. Gastritis
   b. Diverticulitis
   c. Pancreatitis
   d. Cholecystitis

CHAPTER 3 · ANSWERS AND RATIONALES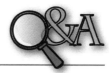

1. The answer is c.

2. The answer is c.

3. The answer is b.

4. The answer is d.

5. The answer is a.

6. The answer is d.

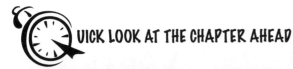
Calcium and phosphorus are required for mineralization of fetal bones and teeth; energy; cell production; and acid-base buffering. Sources of calcium include milk, legumes, nuts, dried fruits, and dark leafy vegetables (kale, cabbage, collards, and turnip greens). Sources of phosphorus include milk, eggs, and meat.

Magnesium is essential for cellular metabolism and structural growth. Sources of magnesium include milk, whole grains, beet greens, nuts, legumes, and tea.

Iron-deficiency anemia decreases the oxygen-carrying capacity of maternal blood, which lowers fetal oxygen levels. A hematocrit below 34% in pregnant women is called **physiologic anemia** of pregnancy.

Iodine deficiency is the most widespread nutritional cause of impaired brain development, cretinism, and mental retardation in newborns.

Sodium is essential for proper metabolism and regulation. Moderate sodium intake from fresh foods is recommended, even for women with pregnancy-induced hypertension or preexisting high blood pressure. Pregnant women should avoid salty or processed foods.

Potassium helps maintain intracellular fluid, serves muscle contractions and transmission of nerve impulses, and assists in regulating blood pressure. Sources of potassium include potatoes, spinach, melons, bananas, fresh meat, milk, coffee, and tea.

4

Nutrition Facts Related to Pregnancy: Minerals

TERMS
- [ ] **physiologic anemia**
- [ ] **iron deficiency anemia**

Zinc is involved in protein metabolism and synthesis of DNA and RNA. A zinc deficiency may affect embryonic growth and cause malformation. Sources of zinc include milk, liver, shellfish, and wheat bran.

CALCIUM AND PHOSPHORUS

Minerals are needed for growth of new tissue. Calcium and phosphorus are involved in the mineralization of fetal bones and teeth, in energy, cell production, and acid-base buffering. (See Appendix A.) Calcium is absorbed and used more effectively during pregnancy.

Minerals are needed for growth of new tissue.

Calcium is absorbed and used more effectively during pregnancy.

Prenatally, teeth begin to form at 8 weeks; 6-year molars calcify at completion of term pregnancy. Bone calcification occurs during the last 2 or 3 months.

If calcium intake is decreased, fetal needs will be met by demineralization of maternal bone. Caffeine increases urinary excretion of calcium; therefore women who consume a large amount of caffeine may need to increase calcium levels.

The DRI for calcium is 1000 mg/day for women over age 19 and 1300 mg/day for younger women (Table 4-1). Sources of calcium include milk, legumes, nuts, dried fruits, and dark green leafy vegetables (kale, cabbage, collards, and turnip greens). The DRI of phosphorus is 700 mg/day for women over the age of 19 and 1250 mg/day for women under age 19. Sources of phosphorus include milk, eggs, and meat.

Sources of calcium include milk, legumes, nuts, dried fruits, and dark green leafy vegetables (kale, cabbage, collards, and turnip greens).

Sources of phosphorus include milk, eggs, and meat.

An excess of phosphorus can result in an unbalanced calcium-phosphorus ratio, resulting in a decreased absorption of calcium and an increased excretion of calcium.

Table 4-1 Sources of Calcium

- Yogurt
- Milk
- Natural cheeses, such as mozzarella, cheddar, Swiss, and Parmesan
- Cereals with added calcium
- Fruit juice with added calcium
- Pudding made with milk
- Soups made with milk
- Dark green leafy vegetables (kale, cabbage, collards, and turnip greens)

Some women may need to limit foods high in phosphorus, such as snack foods, processed meats, and cola drinks.

MAGNESIUM

Pregnant women need to have adequate amounts of magnesium, iron, and vitamin D. Magnesium is essential for cellular metabolism and structural growth. The DRI of magnesium is 400 mg/day for women under age 19, 350 mg/day for women ages 19–30, and 360 mg/day for women 31–50 years old. Sources of magnesium include milk, whole grains, beet greens, nuts, legumes, and tea.

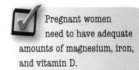
Pregnant women need to have adequate amounts of magnesium, iron, and vitamin D.

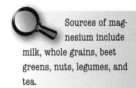
Sources of magnesium include milk, whole grains, beet greens, nuts, legumes, and tea.

IRON

The DRI iron requirement for women during pregnancy is 27 mg/day (Table 4-2). Anemia is mainly caused by low iron stores and/or inadequate intake of Vitamin B_6 and Vitamin B_{12}, folic acid, ascorbic acid, copper, zinc.

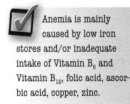
Anemia is mainly caused by low iron stores and/or inadequate intake of Vitamin B_6 and Vitamin B_{12}, folic acid, ascorbic acid, copper, zinc.

Iron-deficiency anemia decreases the oxygen-carrying capacity of maternal blood, which decreases fetal oxygen levels.

Table 4-2 Sources of Iron

- Spinach
- Enriched and whole-grain breads
- Cereals with added iron
- Liver
- Shellfish, such as shrimp and clams
- Kidney beans, black-eyed peas, and lentils

Absorption of iron is generally higher for animal products than for vegetable products, and vitamin C enhances absorption.

The normal hematocrit in nonpregnant women is 38 to 47%. A hematocrit below 34% in pregnant women is referred to as **physiologic anemia** of pregnancy and is the result of the normal expansion of blood volume during pregnancy.

IODINE

The iodine requirement during pregnancy is 220 mcg/day for women. Inorganic iodine is excreted in urine during pregnancy. Enlargement of the thyroid gland may occur if iodine is not replaced by sufficient dietary intake in the form of supplements.

 Iodine deficiency is the most widespread nutritional cause of impaired brain development, cretinism, and mental retardation in newborns.

Sodium is essential for proper metabolism and regulation. A moderate sodium intake of 1.5 g/day is recommended. A pregnant woman should not limit sodium intake even if she has pregnancy-induced hypertension or preexisting high blood pressure. To maintain appropriate sodium levels, it is important for women to eat fresh foods and avoid salty or processed foods.

 To maintain appropriate sodium levels, it is important for women to eat fresh foods and avoid salty or processed foods.

POTASSIUM

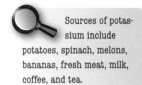

Potassium helps to maintain intracellular fluid and serves as an important component of muscle contractions and transmission of nerve impulses. Potassium also assists in regulating blood pressure. The DRI of potassium during pregnancy is 4.7 g/day. Sources of potassium include potatoes, spinach, melons, bananas, fresh meat, milk, coffee, and tea.

Sources of potassium include potatoes, spinach, melons, bananas, fresh meat, milk, coffee, and tea.

ZINC

The DRI of zinc is 12 mg/day for pregnant 14–18-year-olds and 11 mg/day for 19–50-year-olds. Zinc is involved in protein metabolism and synthesis of DNA and RNA. A zinc deficiency may affect embryonic growth and cause malformation. Sources of zinc include milk, liver, shellfish, and wheat bran.

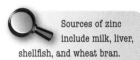

Sources of zinc include milk, liver, shellfish, and wheat bran.

CHAPTER 4 · QUESTIONS

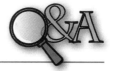

1. During pregnancy, what is the DRI of calcium for women 19 years of age and older?
   a. 1000 mg
   b. 1200 mg
   c. 1500 mg
   d. 1800 mg

2. During pregnancy, what is the DRI of vitamin D?
   a. 10 mcg
   b. 20 mcg
   c. 40 mcg
   d. 50 mcg

3. During pregnancy, what is the DRI of folate?
   a. 200 mcg
   b. 400 mcg
   c. 600 mcg
   d. 800 mcg

4. During pregnancy, what is the DRI of iron for women under the age of 19?
   a. 27 mg
   b. 35 mg
   c. 47 mg
   e. 55 mg

5. The DRI of potassium for women during pregnancy is
   a. 2.7 g/day
   b. 3.0 g/day
   c. 4.7 g/day
   d. 5.0 g/day

CHAPTER 4 • ANSWERS AND RATIONALES

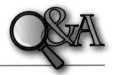

1. The answer is a.

2. The answer is d.

3. The answer is c.

4. The answer is a.

5. The answer is c.

Vitamin A is involved in the growth of epithelial cells; contributes to the metabolism of carbohydrates, fats, and cholesterol; necessary in the synthesis of glycogen; part of the tissue surrounding nerve fibers; and important in the formation and development of eyes during fetal growth. Sources include deep green and yellow vegetables, fruits, liver, liver oil, kidney, egg yolk, cream, butter, and fortified margarine.

Vitamin D is important in the absorption and use of calcium and phosphorus in skeletal development. Sources include fortified milk, margarine, butter, liver, and egg yolks.

Vitamin E is an antioxidant, an essential nutrient for the formation of red blood cells, important in treating muscular pain and intermittent claudication, helps surface healing of wounds and burns, and protects lung tissue from the effects of smog. Sources include vegetable fats and oils, whole grains, greens, eggs, and breast milk.

Vitamin K is essential in the synthesis of prothrombin and its related function in blood clotting. Sources include cheese, egg yolk, liver, and green leafy vegetables.

Vitamin C helps develop connective tissue and the vascular system and is essential in the formation of collagen, which binds cells together. Sources include citrus fruits, tomatoes, cantaloupes, strawberries, potatoes, broccoli, and other leafy green vegetables.

5

Nutrition Facts Related to Pregnancy: Vitamins

TERMS
- [ ] pernicious anemia
- [ ] scurvy
- [ ] pellagra

B-complex vitamins serve as vital coenzyme factors in reactions such as cell respiration, glucose oxidation, and energy metabolism. Sources of thiamine include pork, liver, milk, potatoes, enriched breads, and cereals. Sources of riboflavin include milk, liver, eggs, enriched breads, and cereals.

Niacin works with riboflavin in the cellular coenzyme systems that convert proteins and small amounts of glycerol from fats to glucose and that oxidize glucose to release controlled energy. Sources include meat, fish, poultry, liver, whole grains, enriched breads, cereals, and peanuts.

Folic acid promotes fetal growth and prevents the macrocytic, megaloblastic anemia of pregnancy. Sources include fresh green leafy vegetables, kidney, liver, food yeasts, and peanuts.

Pantothenic acid is an essential constituent of the body's key activating agent, coenzyme A. Sources include meats, egg yolk, legumes, whole-grain cereals, and breads.

Vitamin B_6 is associated with amino acid metabolism. Sources include wheat germ, yeast, fish, liver, pork, potatoes, and lentils.

Vitamin B_{12} deficiencies may result in pernicious anemia. Sources include animal food products such as liver, kidney, lean meat, milk, egg, and cheese.

Vitamins (see Appendix A) are organic substances needed for growth. Vitamins cannot be synthesized by the body in adequate amounts and are grouped according to solubility as described in Chapter 1.

 Megadoses of vitamins, especially vitamins A, D, C, and B$_6$, can have a negative effect on the fetus and can become toxic. Excessive intake of vitamin C may block the body's use of vitamin B$_{12}$.

VITAMIN A

The DRI of vitamin A is 750 mcg/day for women 14–18 years of age and 770 mcg/day for women 19 years of age and older. The blood serum level of vitamin A decreases slightly in early pregnancy, rises in late pregnancy, and falls before the onset of labor. Vitamin A

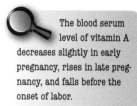
The blood serum level of vitamin A decreases slightly in early pregnancy, rises in late pregnancy, and falls before the onset of labor.

- is involved in the growth of epithelial cells, which are part of the skin and line the gastrointestinal tract.
- contributes to the metabolism of carbohydrates, fats, and cholesterol.
- is necessary in the synthesis of glycogen.
- is part of the tissue surrounding nerve fibers.
- is important in the formation and development of eyes during fetal growth.

 Deficiencies of vitamin A are uncommon and are associated with preterm birth, intrauterine growth retardation, and decreased birth weight. Excessive amounts of vitamin A can cause eye, ear, and bone malformations; cleft palate; possible renal anomalies; and central nervous system (CNS) damage.

Sources of vitamin A include deep green and yellow vegetables, fruits, liver, liver oil, kidney, egg yolk, cream, butter, and fortified margarine.

Sources of vitamin A include deep green and yellow vegetables, fruits, liver, liver oil, kidney, egg yolk, cream, butter, and fortified margarine.

VITAMIN D

The DRI of vitamin D is 5 mcg/day. Vitamin D is important in the absorption and utilization of calcium and phosphorus in skeletal development.

Deficiencies of vitamin D result in reduced fetal bone calcification, hypoplasia of dental enamel, and intrauterine rickets. Excessive intake of vitamin D (usually from a high-potency vitamin preparation) can cause hypercalcemia and cardiac defects (aortic stenosis).

Symptoms of vitamin D toxicity include: excessive thirst, loss of appetite, vomiting, weight loss, irritability, and high blood calcium levels. Sources of vitamin D include fortified milk, margarine, butter, liver, and egg yolks.

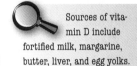

Symptoms of vitamin D toxicity include excessive thirst, loss of appetite, vomiting, weight loss, irritability, and high blood calcium levels.

Sources of vitamin D include fortified milk, margarine, butter, liver, and egg yolks.

VITAMIN E

The DRI of vitamin E is 15 mg/day for pregnant women. The major function of vitamin E is as an antioxidant (takes on oxygen, which prevents chemical changes in another substance). Vitamin E decreases the oxidation of vitamin A in the intestinal tract and the oxidation of polyunsaturated fats.

Vitamin E is an essential nutrient for the synthesis of nucleic acids required in the formation of red blood cells in the bone marrow. It is important in treating certain types of muscular pain and intermittent claudication, in surface healing of wounds and burns, and in protecting lung tissue from the damaging effects of smog. Vitamin E is found in breast milk.

Vitamin E is found in breast milk.

Deficiency symptoms include the long-term inability to absorb fats, particularly in cystic fibrosis, liver cirrhosis, postgastrectomy, obstructive jaundice, pancreatic problems, and sprue. Excessive amounts of vitamin E may lead to abnormal coagulation of blood in the newborn.

Sources of vitamin E include vegetable fats and oils, whole grains, greens, and eggs.

Sources of vitamin E include vegetable fats and oils, whole grains, greens, and eggs.

VITAMIN K

The DRI of vitamin K is 75 mcg/day for pregnant women 14–18 years of age and 90 mcg/day for women over the age of 19. Vitamin K is essential in the synthesis of prothrombin and its related function in blood clotting. The synthesis of vitamin K occurs in the intestinal tract by *Escherichia coli* which normally inhabit the large intestine.

 Vitamin K deficiency may result in malabsorption syndromes or extended use of antibiotics.

Sources of vitamin K include cheese, egg yolk, liver, green leafy vegetables.

 Sources of vitamin K include cheese, egg yolk, liver, green leafy vegetables.

VITAMIN C

The DRI of vitamin C is 80 mg/day for pregnant women 14–18 years of age, and 85 mg/day for women over the age of 19. The major function is development of connective tissue and the vascular system. Vitamin C is essential in the formation of collagen, which binds cells together.

A vitamin C deficiency can reduce collagen, causing cell structure breakdown, muscular weakness, capillary hemorrhage, and eventual death. Maternal megadoses of vitamin C may cause a rebound form of **scurvy**.

Maternal plasma levels of vitamin C progressively decline throughout pregnancy, with values at term about half of midpregnancy level.

Vitamin C appears to concentrate in the placenta, since levels in the fetus are 50% above maternal levels.

Vitamin C is readily destroyed by water and oxidation; thus, foods containing vitamin C require limited exposure to air, heat, and water during storage and cooking. Sources of vitamin C include citrus fruits, tomatoes, cantaloupes, strawberries, potatoes, broccoli, and other leafy green vegetables.

 Maternal plasma levels of vitamin C progressively decline throughout pregnancy, with values at term about half of midpregnancy level.

 Sources of vitamin C include citrus fruits, tomatoes, cantaloupes, strawberries, potatoes, broccoli, and other leafy green vegetables.

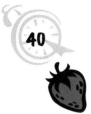

B VITAMIN COMPLEX

The B-complex vitamins serve as vital coenzyme factors in reactions such as cell respiration, glucose oxidation, and energy metabolism. Thiamine has a DRI for pregnant women of 1.4 mg/day. Sources of thiamine include pork, liver, milk, potatoes, enriched breads, cereals.

Sources of thiamine include pork, liver, milk, potatoes, enriched breads, cereals.

The DRI of riboflavin for a pregnant woman is 1.4 mg/day. The lower the protein intake, the higher the riboflavin level. A deficiency of riboflavin is manifested by cheilosis (fissures and excreted cracks of the lips and corners of the mouth) and other skin lesions. Pregnant women may excrete less riboflavin and still require more because of increased energy and protein needs. Sources of riboflavin include milk, liver, eggs, enriched breads, and cereals.

A deficiency of riboflavin is manifested by cheilosis (fissures and excreted cracks of the lips and corners of the mouth) and other skin lesions.

Sources of riboflavin include milk, liver, eggs, enriched breads, and cereals.

Niacin has a DRI for pregnant women of 18 mg/day. Niacin works with riboflavin in the cellular coenzyme systems that convert proteins and a small amount of glycerol from fats to glucose, and that oxidize glucose to release controlled energy.

 A deficiency of niacin produces pellagra, which is characterized by a scaly dermatitis and may have fatal effects on the nervous system.

Symptoms of niacin deficiency include weakness, anorexia, indigestion, skin eruptions. Sources of niacin include meat, fish, poultry, liver, whole grains, enriched breads, cereals, peanuts.

Symptoms of niacin deficiency include weakness, anorexia, indigestion, skin eruptions.

The DRI of folate for pregnant women is 600 mcg/day. Folic acid promotes fetal growth and prevents the macrocytic, megaloblastic anemia of pregnancy, although megaloblastic anemia due to folate deficiency is rarely found in the United States.

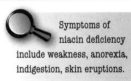

Sources of niacin include meat, fish, poultry, liver, whole grains, enriched breads, cereals, peanuts.

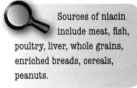

A woman who previously delivered a fetus with a neural tube defect requires supplementation of 4 mg/day at least 1 month before conception and through the first trimester.

 An inadequate intake of folic acid is associated with neural tube defects (e.g., spina bifida, meningomyelocele).

Folic acid is easily destroyed in cooking. Sources of folic acid include fresh green leafy vegetables, kidney, liver, food yeasts, and peanuts.

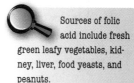
Sources of folic acid include fresh green leafy vegetables, kidney, liver, food yeasts, and peanuts.

OTHER VITAMINS

Pantothenic acid has a DRI for pregnant women of 6 mg/day. Pantothenic acid is an essential constituent of the body's key activating agent, coenzyme A. Sources of pantothenic acid include meats, egg yolk, legumes, whole-grain cereals, and breads.

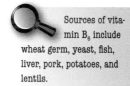
Sources of pantothenic acid include meats, egg yolk, legumes, whole-grain cereals, and breads.

The DRI of vitamin B_6 (pyridoxine) is 1.9 mg/day. Vitamin B_6 is associated with amino acid metabolism. Sources of vitamin B_6 include wheat germ, yeast, fish, liver, pork, potatoes, and lentils.

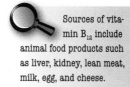
Sources of vitamin B_6 include wheat germ, yeast, fish, liver, pork, potatoes, and lentils.

The DRI of vitamin B_{12} (cobalamin) is 2.6 mcg/day. Vitamin B_{12} can be deficient in women who are vegans.

Vitamin B_{12} deficiencies may result in pernicious anemia.

Sources of vitamin B_{12} include animal food products such as liver, kidney, lean meat, milk, egg, and cheese.

Sources of vitamin B_{12} include animal food products such as liver, kidney, lean meat, milk, egg, and cheese.

CHAPTER 5 · QUESTIONS

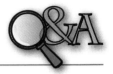

1. Sources of vitamin A include:
   a. Milk and other dairy products
   b. Red meats
   c. Whole grains, vegetable fats, and oils
   d. Deep green and yellow vegetables, liver, and egg yolk

2. Excessive amounts of vitamin E by the pregnant woman may lead to:
   a. Dry skin in the newborn
   b. Abnormal
   c. Telangiectasia
   d. Dry mouth

3. The DRI of vitamin D is:
   a. 3 mcg/day
   b. 4 mcg/day
   c. 5 mcg/day
   d. 7 mcg/day

4. The major function of vitamin _____ is development of connective tissue and the vascular system:
   a. A
   b. B
   c. C
   d. D

5. Sources of riboflavin include:
   a. Breads and cereals
   b. Green leafy vegetables
   c. Red meats
   d. Poultry

CHAPTER 5 · ANSWERS AND RATIONALES

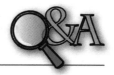

1. The answer is a.

2. The answer is b.

3. The answer is c.

4. The answer is c.

5. The answer is a.

Breastfeeding lessens the incidence of newborn infection, promotes growth in the newborn, and provides immunologic factors to the newborn.

At times, breastfeeding is delayed because of changes in the mother or newborn. The mother then needs to pump her breasts at least five times a day.

Often women choose not to breastfeed based on misinformation.

Breastfeeding requires sufficient fluid intake and nutritional intake.

Breast milk is the ideal food for the first six months.

During pregnancy, a woman should eat as little as possible of dietary cholesterol, trans fatty acids, or saturated fatty acids.

Women do not need to drink milk to make milk. However, adequate fluid intake is essential.

It is recommended that the total caloric intake for lactation be about 2500 to 2700 kcal/day.

6

Lactation

TERMS
- ☐ lactose
- ☐ immunological factors

FACTORS AFFECTING THE DECISION TO BREASTFEED

Women need to have basic information regarding the advantages and disadvantages of breastfeeding before reaching a decision. Relevant factors include body image, sexuality, sexual practices, family traditions, presence of significant others, lifestyle, economics and the need to return to work, and drug and alcohol use.

Breastfeeding lessens the incidence of infection, promotes growth, and provides immunologic factors to the newborn.

TIPS FOR DELAYED BREASTFEEDING

At times, breastfeeding is delayed because of changes in the mother or newborn. In either case, the mother then needs to pump her breasts at least five times a day. A mother should plan breast pumps around the times of visits with the baby. She should pump right before bedtime to ensure at least 6 hours of sleep. It is important for her to keep her breasts stimulated to be ready for feeding.

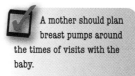

A mother should plan breast pumps around the times of visits with the baby.

Following pumping, breast milk must be stored in sterile, rigid plastic or glass containers. IgA (an immunoglobulin) is destroyed when milk is stored in soft, plastic bag liners.

MATERNAL BEHAVIORS THAT AFFECT LACTATION

Women often choose not to breastfeed based on misinformation (e.g., their breasts are too small; no one in their family was successful). Some women desire immediate weight loss and choose not to breastfeed. Some women are lactose intolerant.

WAYS TO ENHANCE LACTATION

Women should be encouraged to eat a variety of foods, but avoid foods that are not tolerated well by her or the newborn. Breastfeeding requires sufficient fluid intake and nutritional intake. Women need to look for ways to maintain breastfeeding within their lifestyle. Support groups provide valuable information.

NUTRITION FACTS

Breastmilk is the ideal food for the first 6 months of an infant's life. A mother who is a vegetarian and has no intake of animal products requires a vitamin B_{12} supplement during pregnancy and lactation. Recommendations for breastfeeding are listed in Appendix A.

- The DRI for protein needs is 71 g/day.
- The DRI for carbohydrates is 210 g/day.
- No DRI has been established for dietary cholesterol, trans fatty acids, or saturated fatty acids during pregnancy. Women are encouraged to eat as little as possible of them, while consuming a nutritionally adequate diet.

MINERALS

The DRI for calcium during lactation is 1300 mg/d for women ages 14–18 and 1000 mg/d for women 19 years and older. This is not more than is needed during pregnancy since the amount of calcium used for fetal skeletal development is then used for milk production. The DRI for phosphorus for women under 18 years is 1250 mg/d and for women 18 years and older it is 700 mg/d.

Iron requirements for women ages 14–18 are 10 mg/day; for women over age 19.9 mg/day. The DRI for fluoride is 3 mg/day.

VITAMINS

The DRI for vitamin C is 115 mg/day for women ages 14–18, and 120 mg/day for women over 19. There is an increased need for vitamin A (1200 mcg/day at ages 14–18; 1300 mcg/day at ages 19–50), and B complex (thiamine, 1.4 mg/day; niacin, 17 mg/day; B_6, 2 mg/day; and B_{12}, 2.8 mcg/day). The requirement for vitamin D is 5 mcg/day.

FLUIDS

Women do not need to drink milk to make milk. However, adequate fluid intake is essential. If fluid intake is insufficient, urine will be concentrated (dark yellow), and there is potential for constipation.

CALORIES

It is recommended that the kcal increase for lactation be 500 kcal more than the usual adult allowance. The daily total is about 2500 to 2700 kcal.

Questions to Ask the Mother

What have you eaten in the last 24 hours?

What is your normal weight pattern?

What is your normal pattern of food intake?

What type (if any) of vitamin and mineral supplements do you take?

Do you have any food allergies or intolerances?

Do you have family members or friends who have breast-fed their children?

Have you breast-fed any of your other children?

What are the cultural influences on your dietary intake?

CHAPTER 6 · QUESTIONS

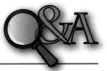

1. What is the recommended daily kilocaloric (kcal) increase for lactation?
   a. 500 kcal
   b. 550 kcal
   c. 600 kcal
   d. 650 kcal

2. In cases where breastfeeding is delayed, a woman needs to pump her breasts for 10 minutes how many times each day (at least)?
   a. 2
   b. 3
   c. 4
   d. 5

3. Breast milk is considered the ideal food for the first how many months of life?
   a. 2
   b. 4
   c. 6
   d. 8

4. During lactation, what is the standard DRI for calcium per day for women 19 years and older?
   a. 1000 mg
   b. 1200 mg
   c. 1500 mg
   d. 1800 mg

5. What is the DRI of protein per day for lactating women?
   a. 40 g
   b. 55 g
   c. 60 g
   d. 71 g

6. What is the DRI for phosphorus for the lactating woman under 18 years?
   a. 1055 mg/day
   b. 1255 mg/day
   c. 1455 mg/day
   d. 1555 mg/day

7. What is the DRI for vitamin C for the lactating woman 19 to 50 years?
   a. 50 mg/day
   b. 70 mg/day
   c. 100 mg/day
   d. 120 mg/day

8. What is the DRI for iron for lactating women over 19 years?
   a. 9 mg/day
   b. 10 mg/day
   c. 14 mg/day
   d. 16 mg/day

9. What is the DRI for vitamin D in lactating women over 19 years?
   a. 3 mg/day
   b. 5 mg/day
   c. 7 mg/day
   d. 9 mg/day

10. What is the DRI for vitamin B_{12} for lactating women over 19 years?
    a. 2 mg/day
    b. 2.2 mg/day
    c. 2.4 mg/day
    d. 2.8 mg/day

CHAPTER 6 • ANSWERS AND RATIONALES

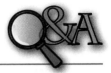

1. The answer is a.

2. The answer is b.

3. The answer is c.

4. The answer is a.

5. The answer is c.

6. The answer is b.

7. The answer is d.

8. The answer is a.

9. The answer is b.

10. The answer is d.

The volume of fluid intake increases from 10–15 mL per feeding in the first 24 hours to 60–90 mL per feeding over the first few days.

Colostrum is the initial breast secretion that contains sufficient calories, nutrients, macrophages, and antibodies necessary for the newborn.

Mothers should be reminded to have the newborn latch onto the entire areola, not just the nipple.

Commercially prepared formula is recommended for bottle-fed newborns and infants during the first 6–12 months. Low-fat (2%) milk, commercial milk substitutes, and dry milk are not recommended for infants less than 1 year old.

Before preparing formula, the caregiver should wash hands, the top of the can, and all related equipment with warm, soapy water, and rinse well. Opened cans of formula should be stored in a covered container (not the can) and refrigerated and used within 48 hours.

There are several types of formula. Solutions of high osmolarity may draw water into the small intestine, causing diarrhea and possible dehydration and electrolyte imbalance. Cow's milk is unmodified and not suitable for newborns.

The decision to breast-feed depends on the stability of the newborn, and the mother's condition. If the woman desires to breast-feed but it is not feasible, the mother may need to pump her breasts and store milk for later use. In some cases, the mother may pump her breasts and the breast

7

The Newborn (Birth–4 Weeks): Part I

TERMS
- [ ] latch
- [ ] bonding
- [ ] milk modifiers
- [ ] colostrum

milk is given via a nasogastric tube or by bottle with a special nipple to reduce the energy demands of breastfeeding.

To create a positive feeding experience, the newborn should suck a pacifier during gavage. This may make the transition to nipple feeding easier. The criteria for nipple feeding include coordinated sucking, swallowing, and breathing; adequate gag reflex; unlabored sucking; and steady weight gain.

PATTERNS OF GROWTH FOR FULL-TERM NEWBORNS

Most newborns experience 5–7% weight loss during the first few days of life. However, full-term newborns usually regain the initial weight loss within 10–14 days. Newborns will continue to gain approximately 1 oz/day until they have doubled their weight in 6 months. A newborn's length will double during the first year. (Refer to Table 7-1 for the average physical parameters of the newborn.)

During the first 24 hours, the newborn adjusts to extrauterine life and the digestive system is cleared of meconium. The volume of fluid intake increases from 10–15 mL/feeding in the first 24 hours to 60–90 mL/feeding over the first few days. The volume capacity requires frequent feedings of the newborn.

Common Patterns of Eating

Breastfeeding
Colostrum is the initial breast secretion that contains sufficient calories, nutrients, macrophages, and antibodies necessary for the newborn. The amount and temperature of the milk are suitable for the newborn until mature breast milk is available within a few days.

Table 7-1 Physical Parameters of a Newborn

Length, 19–21 in (48–53 cm)
Weight, 6–9 lbs (2700–4000 g); average, 7.5 lb (3400 g)

It is important for mothers to use the breastfeeding experience as an opportunity to relax and enjoy the baby so the time spent is stress-reducing not stress-producing. It is very important for mothers when breastfeeding to be sure to maintain nutrition and fluid requirements as well as to schedule rests and adequate sleep.

> It is important for mothers to use the breastfeeding experience as an opportunity to relax and enjoy the baby so the time spent is stress-reducing not stress-producing.

Mothers need to be reminded to have the newborn **latch** on to the entire areola, not just the nipple. Otherwise, the milk is not expressed successfully and the baby becomes frustrated and cries. All of this produces anxiety between the newborn and the mother, frequently resulting in poor nutritional intake. Mothers who do not have adequate support and education may discontinue breastfeeding because of the poor quality of the interaction.

Bottle-feeding

Commercially prepared formula is recommended for bottle-fed newborns and infants during the first 6–12 months.

> Commercially prepared formula is recommended for bottle-fed newborns and infants during the first 6–12 months.

Questions to Ask the Mother

If Breastfeeding:

How many minutes are you feeding the baby with each breast?

How frequently are you breastfeeding?

Does the baby seem satisfied?

How many diapers are saturated with urine each day?

How many bowel movements is the baby having each day?

What are the characteristics of the stool?

What are the baby's responses to feeding?

If Bottle-Feeding:

How frequently are you feeding the baby?

How much does the baby drink?

Does the baby seem satisfied?

How many diapers are saturated with urine each day?

How many bowel movements is the baby having each day?

What are the characteristics of the stool?

What are the baby's responses to feeding?

Prepared formulas are available in ready-to-use, concentrated, or powdered preparations. They must meet the infant's need for water, energy, vitamins, and minerals and must be readily digestible. The caregiver needs to compare formulas, as they vary in protein, fat, and carbohydrate content.

Dry milk is not recommended for infants <1 year old because it provides an excessive intake of protein with inadequate calories. This causes mobilization of body fat for energy requirements and growth needs. Dry milk also lacks an adequate content of iron, ascorbic acid, and essential fatty acids.

Low-fat (2%) milk and commercial milk substitutes are also not recommended for newborns or infants because they may not provide adequate nutritional intake.

Prior to preparing the formula, it is important for the caregiver to wash his or her hands, wash the top of the can, and wash all related equipment with warm, soapy water and rinse well with hot water (if applicable). Opened cans of formula should be stored in a covered container (not the can) and refrigerated and used within 48 hours.

> Prior to preparing the formula, it is important for the caregiver to wash his or her hands, wash the top of the can, and wash all related equipment with warm, soapy water and rinse well with hot water (if applicable).

Most ready-to-feed formulas are 20 kcal/oz. Standards for minimum levels of 29 nutrients and maximum levels for 9 are set by the American Academy of Pediatrics.

There are several types of formula preparation, including ready-to-feed liquids, concentrated liquids, powdered forms (which need to be mixed with water), and evaporated milk. (Evaporated milk formula consists of mixing 13 oz. of evaporated milk, plus 19½ oz. of water, and 3 tablespoons of sugar or commercially processed corn syrup. Vitamin C and iron are added.)

Additional important considerations regarding formulas include stability and osmolarity. Formulas are mixtures of emulsified fats, proteins, carbohydrates, vitamins, minerals, and thickening or stabilizing agents. They are designed to prevent separation of the components and to add stability for a longer shelf life.

 Solutions of high osmolarity may draw water into the small intestine, causing diarrhea and possible dehydration and electrolyte imbalance.

Cow's milk is unmodified and is not suitable for newborns. Several problems with
the use of cow's milk include gastrointestinal
bleeding; a renal solute load that is too great

> ✓ Cow's milk is
> unmodified and is not
> suitable for newborns.

for the infant's renal system, causing possible dehydration; and iron states
(high calcium and phosphorus levels that inhibit iron absorption).

PRETERM NEWBORNS (BORN BEFORE 37 WEEKS) AND LOW-BIRTH-WEIGHT NEWBORNS

High-risk newborns are susceptible to water
loss due to a high surface to body mass ratio,
permeable skin, the use of radiant warm-
ers and phototherapy, and urinary and
fecal excretion. The decision to breast-feed
depends on the stability of the newborn, the
reasons for early delivery, and the mother's
condition. If desired and feasible, breastfeeding is initiated once the premature
reaches 34–35 weeks. If the mother desires
to breast-feed but it is not feasible, she may
need to pump her breasts and store milk for
later use.

> ✓ High-risk newborns
> are susceptible to
> water loss due to a high
> surface to body mass ratio,
> permeable skin, the use of
> radiant warmers and pho-
> totherapy, and urinary and
> fecal excretion.

> 🔍 The decision
> to breast-feed
> depends on the stability of
> the newborn, the reasons
> for early delivery, and the
> mother's condition.

In some cases, the mother may pump
her breasts and the breast milk is given via
a nasogastric tube or by bottle with a special nipple to reduce the energy
demands of breastfeeding.

Preterm breast milk has adequate immunological properties but is
low in calcium and phosphorus; in some cases, an additive (in liquid or
powder) known as a *milk modifier* is used to modify the deficiencies.

Several factors (fluid intake and output, body weight changes, urine
specific gravity and osmolarity, serum electrolyte and creatinine concentrations, and blood urea nitrogen [BUN]) determine fluid replacement.

Preterm infant formulas have been modified to provide adequate calories, carbohydrate changes to give lower osmolarity, and fat modifications to promote absorption.

In some cases, the mother may not be able to participate regularly in
feeding the newborn. She may be discharged before the newborn or she

is unable to participate regularly in feeding the newborn because of her schedule (responsibilities of work, home, and other children). Also, the presence of maternal risk factors such as pregnancy-induced hypertension, chronic hypertension, gestational diabetes, and type 2 diabetes mellitus may affect the mother's decision to breast-feed or bottle-feed, and the level of her participation.

Preterm newborns are at greater risk for infection, failure to thrive syndrome, and additional complications than are full-term babies. Preterm newborns and infants have special feeding considerations. They often have uncoordinated sucking and swallowing. Preterm newborns also are at risk for incompetent cardiac sphincter, delayed gastric emptying time, decreased absorption of fat, incomplete digestion of protein, and decreased or uncoordinated motility. To create a positive feeding experience, the newborn can suck a pacifier during gavage. This may make the transition to nipple feeding easier. The criteria for nipple feeding include coordinated sucking, swallowing, and breathing; adequate gag reflex (present at 34–36 weeks' gestation); respiratory function that allows unlabored sucking (< 60 breaths/min); and steady weight gain.

> Preterm newborns are at greater risk for infection, failure to thrive syndrome, and additional complications than are full-term babies.

CHAPTER 7 • QUESTIONS

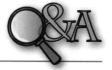

1. Newborns experience how much weight loss during the first few days of life?
   a. 3–5%
   b. 5–7%
   c. 7–9%
   d. 9–10%

2. After the first 24 hours of life, the newborn's stomach capacity of fluid gradually increases to what average number?
   a. 10–15 mL
   b. 20–25 mL
   c. 60–90 mL
   d. 100–125 mL

3. What is the name for the initial breast secretion produced by the postpartum woman?
   a. Breast milk
   b. Colostrum
   c. Galactorrhea
   d. Meconium

4. Commercially prepared formula is recommended for newborns and infants during the first _____ of life.
   a. 3–6 months
   b. 6–12 months
   c. 12–18 months
   d. 18–24 months

5. Dry milk is not recommended for infants less than 1 year because it provides an excessive intake of protein with:
   a. A high intake of fats
   b. Inadequate calories
   c. An excessive amount of iron
   d. A large amount of ascorbic acid

6. If desired and feasible, breastfeeding for newborns who are born before 37 weeks' gestation can begin at what gestation age?
    a. 31–32 weeks
    b. 32–34 weeks
    c. 34–35 weeks
    d. 36–37 weeks

7. What product can be added to eliminate the deficiencies, such as calcium and phosphorus, in preterm breast milk?
    a. Formula
    b. Milk modifier
    c. Dry powdered milk
    d. Mature donor breast milk

8. What criterion for nipple feeding of preterm newborns is included with the criteria of coordinated sucking, swallowing, breathing, and an adequate gag reflex?
    a. Absence of colic
    b. Steady weight gain
    c. Stomach capacity of 90 mL
    d. Presence of the rooting reflex

9. Which of the following maternal risk factors may affect the mother's decision to breast-feed?
    a. Gestational diabetes
    b. Type 2 diabetes
    c. Chronic hypertension
    d. All of the above.

10. High-risk newborns are susceptible to water loss due to:
    a. Urinary and fecal excretion
    b. Excessive perspiration
    c. Low surface to body mass ratio
    d. Nonpermeable skin

CHAPTER 7 · ANSWERS AND RATIONALES

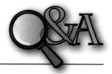

1. **The answer is b.** Less than 5–7% is too little and greater than this amount would be excessive.

2. **The answer is c.**

3. **The answer is b.**

4. **The answer is b.**

5. **The answer is b.** This causes mobilization of body fat for energy requirements and growth needs.

6. **The answer is c.**

7. **The answer is b.**

8. **The answer is b.**

9. **The answer is d.** All may affect the mother's decision and her level of participation.

10. **The answer is a.** The newborn has high surface to body mass ratio; the newborn does not perspire; newborn has high surface to body mass ratio and permeable skin.

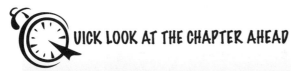

QUICK LOOK AT THE CHAPTER AHEAD

Create a relaxed environment during feeding, and review and record the interactions between the newborn and caregiver during the feeding experience.

The newborn's sleep-wake cycle frequently causes sleep deprivation for the primary care-taker, which can affect the mother-newborn interaction and influence the nutritional intake of the newborn.

Coordination of reflexes, such as the gag, sucking, and swallowing reflexes, facilitates nutritional intake.

The extrusion reflex, which fades by the age of 4 months, does not indicate food preference. When solid foods are fed, placing the food past the tip of the tongue may lessen the reflex.

Provide a routine for eating, preferably when support people are available to help.

Carbohydrates provide 40–45% of total calories in the newborn diet. Lactose is the primary carbohydrate in human milk until the age of 6 months. The advantages of lactose include easy absorption.

Calcium is needed for the rapid bone mineralization that takes place during growth.

Iron from enriched cereals, eggs, and (later) meats is essential for hemoglobin formation.

It is important to watch for signs and symptoms of excessive amounts of vitamin A and vitamin D.

8

The Newborn: Part II

TERMS
☐ reflexes
☐ sleep/wake cycles
☐ lactose

> If the newborn is breastfeeding, it is important to ensure intake of vitamin K (immediately after birth), iron, and fluoride.
>
> If the newborn is bottle-feeding, special formulas for older infants are unnecessary.

BEHAVIORS THAT AFFECT NEWBORN NUTRITION

Common questions to ask the mother or caregiver that impact the newborn's nutrition are listed at the end of the chapter It is very important to consider the interaction between the newborn and caregiver during the feeding experience. One tip is to create a relaxed environment during feeding that can be enhanced with soothing music. It is also helpful to review basic information with the caregiver such as

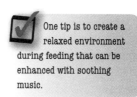

One tip is to create a relaxed environment during feeding that can be enhanced with soothing music.

- proper positioning of the newborn during and after feeding
- the mother's diet if she is breastfeeding
- the newborn's diet in terms of type and amount, and the feeding schedule
- characteristics of the baby's stool
- how the caregiver intervenes when an episode of colic begins, and when the episodes occur over a 24-hour period.

The caregiver can record this information in a diary so that the information reported later is accurate.

The **sleep-wake cycle** of the newborn is related to factors that change throughout the course of infancy. Newborns usually eat every 3–4 hours, which usually sets the initial sleep-wake cycle. The pattern of feeding interaction between the mother and the newborn and the physical environment of the newborn can create different patterns of sleeping.

The newborn's sleep-wake cycle frequently causes sleep deprivation for the primary caretaker, usually the mother. Maternal sleep deprivation can lead to behaviors such as anxiety and depression, which affect the mother-newborn interaction and influence the nutritional intake of the newborn.

Coordination of **reflexes**, such as gagging, sucking, and swallowing, facilitates nutritional intake. These reflexes are part of the criteria for initiating oral feeding in the newborn.

The rooting reflex occurs when the newborn turns toward a stimulus to eat. The caregiver should gently stroke the lips and cheek of the newborn, but only on one side. A baby given multiple stimuli will show confusion and anxiety, and nutritional intake may lessen. The rooting reflex disappears at the age of 3–4 months.

Extrusion is a forward-thrusting movement of the tongue. The extrusion reflex does not indicate food preference. Also, when solid foods are added, placing the food past the tip of the tongue may lessen the reflex. Extrusion fades by the age of 4 months.

WAYS TO ENHANCE NUTRITION

It is very important to provide a routine for eating. Plan eating when support people are available to help (e.g., to help with feeding older children). The caregiver needs to ensure that the time devoted to eating is not stressful and is an opportunity to give total attention to the newborn. Caregivers need to recognize feeding cues (e.g., bringing hand to mouth, rooting reflex, mouthing, sucking). Positioning of the newborn during eating is important and should facilitate eye contact between the child and caregiver.

NUTRITION FACTS

Newborn energy requirements depend on the basal energy requirement for metabolic function; the energy needed for physical activity and digestion of food; and the energy needed for growth (see Appendixes A and B).

> ✓ Newborn energy requirements depend on the basal energy requirement for metabolic function; the energy needed for physical activity and digestion of food; and the energy needed for growth (see Appendixes A and B).

Carbohydrates

The newborn has hepatic glycogen stores; thus, carbohydrates provide 40–45% of total calories in the diet. Newborns have limited ability for gluconeogenesis (formation of glucose) from amino acids and other substrates, and for ketogenesis (formation of ketone bodies from fat), which are mechanisms that provide alternative energy sources.

Lactose is the primary carbohydrate in human milk until the age of 6 months. The advantages of lactose include easy absorption; slower breakdown and absorption may increase calcium absorption.

Minerals

Calcium is needed for the rapid bone mineralization that takes place during growth. At this point, only central sections of the large bones are mineralized. During this time, there is an increased need for calcium for developing teeth, muscle contraction, nerve irritability, blood coagulation, and heart muscle action.

Iron is essential for hemoglobin formation. The fetal store of iron is diminished 4–6 months after birth. Dietary intake should include enriched cereal, eggs, and (later) meats.

Vitamins

It is important to watch for signs and symptoms of excessive amounts of vitamin A: anorexia, slow growth, dryness and cracking of the skin, and enlargement of the liver and spleen.

Vitamin D intake also needs to be monitored for excessive amounts, demonstrated by symptoms such as diarrhea, weight loss, polyuria, and eventual calcification of soft tissues (e.g., renal tubules, blood vessels, bronchi, stomach, and heart).

If the newborn is breastfeeding, it is important to ensure intake of the following supplements:

- Vitamin K is given immediately after birth; iron and fluoride.
- Infants from birth to 6 months require 0.27 mg/day of iron (DRI).
- The DRI of iron increases to 11 mg/day for infants 7 to 12 months (greater than 13 pounds, but less than 20 pounds).
- The DRI for vitamin D at 0–12 months is 5 mcg per day.
- The DRI for fluoride at 0-6 months is 0.01 mg/day and at 7–12 months is 0.5 mg/day.

If the newborn is bottle-feeding, special formulas for older infants are unnecessary.

Questions to Ask the Mother

Have you noticed any rashes on the baby's skin?

What is the baby's sleeping pattern?

What is the baby's total weight gain?

What are the baby's patterns of activity?

Did you participate in routine prenatal care?

Did you have any complications such as gestational hypertension, diabetes mellitus, or gestational diabetes mellitus?

Did youhave any risk factors related to substance abuse (drugs, alcohol, nicotine, caffeine)?

CHAPTER 8 · QUESTIONS

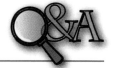

1. What is the term for the forward tongue-thrusting reflex in the newborn?
   a. Rooting reflex
   b. Babinski reflex
   c. Extrusion reflex
   d. Letdown reflex

2. Which mineral is needed for rapid bone mineralization?
   a. Iron
   b. Calcium
   c. Potassium
   d. Magnesium

3. For infants who are born at term, human milk is most desirable for the first:
   a. 2 months
   b. 4 months
   c. 6 months
   d. 12 months

4. If an infant receives commercially prepared formula, it is important to check and see if the contents have been fortified with what?
   a. Calcium and vitamin D
   b. Fluoride and iron
   c. Sodium and potassium
   d. Magnesium and sulfur

5. Carbohydrates provide what amount of calories in the newborn's diet?
   a. 20–30%
   b. 40–45%
   c. 45–50%
   d. 50–55%

6. The storage of fetal iron diminishes after birth during which of the following time periods?
   a. 1–2 months
   b. 2–3 months
   c. 4–6 months
   d. 7–8 months

7. A new mother tells the nurse that she feeds her 8 month old infant carrots three times a day. What's the potential outcome?
   a. The infant will not develop taste buds
   b. Vitamin D toxicity in the infant
   c. The infant will develop visual problems
   d. Vitamin A toxicity in the infant

8. Coordination of reflexes, such as gagging, sucking, and swallowing, is necessary for which of the following?
   a. Initiating oral feeding of the newborn
   b. Decreasing respiratory effort
   c. To aide in the digestive process
   d. To develop socialization skills

9. In a woman who is breast-feeding, the DRI of iron for the infant is?
   a. 9 mg/day
   b. 10 mg/day
   c. 11 mg/day
   d. 12 mg/day

10. Excessive amounts of this vitamin causes diarrhea, weight loss, polyaria, and eventual calcification of soft tissues (e.g., renal tubules):
   a. Vitamin D
   b. Vitamin K
   c. Vitamin E
   d. Vitamin A

CHAPTER 8 • ANSWERS AND RATIONALES

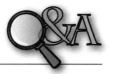

1. The answer is c.

2. The answer is b.

3. The answer is c.

4. The answer is b.

5. The answer is b.

6. The answer is c.

7. The answer is d.

8. The answer is a.

9. The answer is c.

10. The answer is a.

Full-term infants receiving breast milk from a well-nourished mother require no specific vitamins or minerals. From 0 to 6 months, infants should receive 0.01 mg of fluoride and 0.27 mg of iron. If commercially prepared formula is used, it is important to make sure it is fortified with fluoride and iron.

Infants should not be given unmodified whole milk, low-fat milk, or imitation milk because it may contain insufficient calories and nutrients. Whole milk can cause iron deficiency.

Breast milk alone is sufficient for the first 6 months. Low-fat milk is not appropriate for infants and children under the age of 2. There is no nutritional need for solid foods before the baby is 4–6 months old.

The infant should be gradually introduced to and fed a variety of solid foods. Juice can be substituted for one milk feeding. The first foods must be liquid and semiliquid until teeth come in.

Choose foods with appropriate levels of iron, zinc, and calcium.

Infants require more water relative to their size, compared to adults, to manage renal excretion.

9

The Infant (1–12 Months)

TERMS
- ☐ fluoride
- ☐ iron
- ☐ solid foods

For infants born at term, human milk is most desirable for the first 6 months. Full-term infants receiving breast milk from a well-nourished mother require no specific vitamins or minerals. At the ages of 0–6 months, it is recommended that infants receive 0.01 mg of fluoride and 0.27 mg of iron.

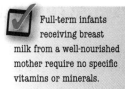
Full-term infants receiving breast milk from a well-nourished mother require no specific vitamins or minerals.

If commercially prepared formula is used, it is important to make sure it is fortified with fluoride and iron. Infants need the fat content in milk and other foods. Infants should not be given unmodified whole milk, low-fat milk, or imitation milk because it may contain insufficient calories and nutrients. Whole milk can cause iron deficiency due to occult gastrointestinal blood loss during infancy.

BEHAVIORS THAT AFFECT NUTRITION

As mentioned in Chapter 8, behaviors such as colic and disturbances in the infant sleep-wake pattern have an impact on the primary caregiver, ultimately creating depression and anxiety in some individuals. During infancy, the central psychosocial goal is to establish a sense of trust as opposed to mistrust. For the infant, food is a way of gaining satisfaction and exploring the environment. Trust is a critical issue; the needs of the infant, such as feeding, touching, and holding in a relaxed environment, must be met consistently. (Refer to Table 9-1.)

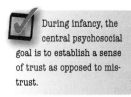
During infancy, the central psychosocial goal is to establish a sense of trust as opposed to mistrust.

Table 9-1 Common Behaviors That Affect Nutritional Intake

- Colic
- Regurgitation
- Caregiver anxiety

By 6 months infant can:
- Feed self a cracker
- Hold bottle

By 12 months infant can:
- Drink from a cup
- Feed self finger foods
- Use a spoon for eating

WAYS TO ENHANCE NUTRITION

It is important to provide the newborn with a routine for eating. The rooting reflex orients the infant to the source of food, which can facilitate nutritional intake. If the mother is breast feeding, she needs to be sure that the baby's mouth is on the areola and not just the nipple. She should allow the baby to nurse 5–10 minutes at each breast and schedule feedings every 3 or 4 hours.

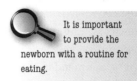

It is important to provide the newborn with a routine for eating.

Initially, the mother needs to change the baby's position with each feeding to ensure that her nipples do not become sore or irritated, leading to a disruption in skin integrity. For some mothers, nipple soreness or irritation causes them to discontinue breastfeeding.

When the mother decides to start weaning the infant from breast feeding, she can substitute one breast-feeding with a bottle-feeding. If weaning the baby from bottle-feeding, the caregiver may start with substituting one bottle-feeding at a time with a cup feeding.

TRANSITION TO SOLID FOODS

There is no nutritional need to give infants solid foods before they are 4–6 months old. Delay of solid foods has the following advantages: It lessens the incidence of allergies; the protrusion reflex fades, making feeding less difficult; the gastrointestinal tract is more mature to handle complex foods; and head control is better developed. Voluntary grasping allows the infant to pick up finger foods, which encourages self-feeding. The development of muscular coordination involving the tongue and swallowing reflex allows semisolid foods to be added. Introduction of solid foods begins with cereal with a little milk, then fruits, vegetables, eggs, potatoes, and meats. Offer solids before milk.

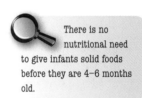

There is no nutritional need to give infants solid foods before they are 4–6 months old.

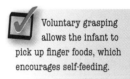

Voluntary grasping allows the infant to pick up finger foods, which encourages self-feeding.

A good schedule to introduce a new food is every 4–7 days, in small amounts. An average amount to give is 1–2 tablespoons at a time. Remember to use small spoons and place the food on the back of the tongue.

As the amount of solid food is increased, the amount of milk given should be decreased to prevent overfeeding.

 Do not mix food in a bottle with a large hole in the nipple and use it to feed the infant, which may cause aspiration, and have a negative effect on eating patterns.

Gradually introduce and feed the infant a variety of foods. It is essential to pay attention to the baby's appetite, to avoid overfeeding and underfeeding. Cereals (rice, barley, oatmeal, high protein) should be fortified with iron (7 mg of iron/3 tablespoons).

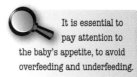
It is essential to pay attention to the baby's appetite, to avoid overfeeding and underfeeding.

Fruit juices should contain vitamin C such as orange juice. The caregiver can substitute juice for one milk feeding.

 Avoid apple, pear, prune, sweet cherry, peach, and grape juices, as they can cause diarrhea or bloating. Do not warm the juice because this destroys the vitamin C content.

NUTRITION FACTS

As mentioned, breast milk alone is sufficient for the first 6 months (see Appendix A). During the first 6 months, the DRI of vitamin K is 2.0 mcg/day; the DRI of iron is 0.27 mg/day; the DRI of fluoride is 0.01 mg/day. From 7 to 12 months, the DRI of vitamin K is 2.5 mcg/day; the DRI of iron is 11 mg/day; and the DRI of fluoride is 0.5 mg/day.

 Low-fat milk is not appropriate for infants and children under the age of 2. Be careful of foods that have high fiber.

Sugar is necessary in moderation. Sodium is necessary in moderation as it helps to control fluid balance.

Choose foods with appropriate levels of iron, zinc, and calcium. Infants who have decreased iron levels are at risk for anemia, abnormal cognitive and social development, and delayed balance, coordination, and motor skills. Decreased zinc levels may lead to decreased immune function and growth. Decreased calcium interferes with normal rapid bone development.

Infancy is a period of rapid growth with high energy requirements (Tables 9-2 and 9-3).

Infants have the ability to digest and absorb proteins, moderate amounts of fat, and simple carbohydrates. They have some difficulty with starch because the starch-splitting enzyme amylase is present only in small amounts. Infants require more water relative to their size, compared to adults, to manage renal excretion. (Refer to Table 9-4.)

 Infancy is a period of rapid growth with high energy requirements (Tables 9-2 and 9-3).

Infants require more water relative to their size, compared to adults, to manage renal excretion.

The first teeth erupt around the age of 4 months, so initial foods must be liquid and semiliquid.

Infants have limited nutritional stores and require supplemental vitamins.

Table 9-2 Infant Parameters and Requirements

Physical Parameters

Length

By age 1 year, birth length has doubled. 1 in. (2.5 cm)/month for the first 6 months and approximately 0.5 in. (1.25 cm) for the next 6 months.

Weight

By age 1 year, infant's weight has tripled [average of 21.5 lb (9.75 kg)]. 1.5 lb (680 g)/month for the first 5 months, then decreases during second half of year.

Energy Requirements

During the first 4 months of life:

50–60% of infant's energy expended for basal metabolism.

10–15% of infant's energy expended for activity.

25–40% of infant's energy expended for growth.

Energy Requirements:

650 kcal/kg for the first 6 months

850 kcal/kg for the next 6 months

Table 9-3 Nutritional Requirements

- Breast milk desirable for the first 6 months.
- Infant consumes about 3–4 oz of formula/feeding for the first 2 months.
- During the first 2 months the infant has approximately 6–8 feedings per day.

Table 9-4 Diet

CHO	0 to 6 months = 60 grams/day
	7 to 12 months = 95 grams/day
Fats	0 to 6 months = 31 grams/day
	7 to 12 months = 30 grams/day
Protein	0 to 6 months = 9.1 grams/day
	7 to 12 months = 11 grams/day
Water	0 to 6 months = 0.7 liters/day
	7 to 12 months = 0.8 liters/day

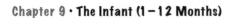

Questions to Ask the Mother

If Breastfeeding

How many minutes does the baby feed at each breast?

How frequently are you breastfeeding?

Does the baby seem satisfied?

How many diapers are saturated with urine each day?

How many bowel movements is the baby having each day?

What are the characteristics of the stool?

What are the baby's responses to feeding?

If Bottle-Feeding

How frequently are you feeding the baby?

How much does the baby drink?

Does the baby seem satisfied?

How many diapers are saturated with urine each day?

How many bowel movements is the baby having each day?

What are the characteristics of the stool?

What are the baby's responses to feeding?

Have there been rashes on the baby's skin?

What is the sleeping pattern of the baby?

What is the total weight gain?

What are the baby's patterns of activity?

What was the prenatal care compliance?

Did you have any complications, such as gestational hypertension, diabetes mellitus, or gestational diabetes?

Did you have any risk factors related to substance abuse (drugs, alcohol, nicotine, caffeine)?

CHAPTER 9 • QUESTIONS

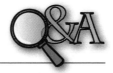

1. During infancy, the essential psychosocial goal is to establish a sense of what?
   a. Identity versus role diffusion
   b. Initiative versus guilt
   c. Trust versus mistrust
   d. Autonomy versus shame and doubt

2. Infants should begin to receive solid foods at what age?
   a. 2–4 months
   b. 4–6 months
   c. 6–8 months
   d. 8–12 months

3. How often should a new solid food be introduced to the infant?
   a. 2–3 days
   b. 3–4 days
   c. 4–7 days
   d. 7–10 days

4. What is an average amount of food to be fed to an infant?
   a. 1–2 tablespoons
   b. 2–4 tablespoons
   c. 4–6 tablespoons
   d. 6–8 tablespoons

5. The recommended amount of iron in iron-fortified cereal is:
   a. 5 mg of iron/3 tablespoons
   b. 6 mg of iron/3 tablespoons
   c. 7 mg of iron/3 tablespoons
   d. 8 mg of iron/3 tablespoons

6. The DRI for vitamin D for infants up to one year is:
   a. 20 µg/day
   b. 15 µg/day
   c. 10 µg/day
   d. 5 µg/day

7. For most infants, the first teeth erupt at what age?
   a. 2 months
   b. 4 months
   c. 6 months
   d. 8 months

8. What is the DRI for iron for infants 7 months to 1 year?
   a. 11 mg/day
   b. 12 mg/day
   c. 13 mg/day
   d. 14 mg/day

9. The mother should allow the newborn to breast-feed for how many minutes at each breast?
   a. 5-10 minutes
   b. 11-20 minutes
   c. 10-15 minutes
   d. 15-20 minutes

10. Which of the following juices should a mother select for her infant?
   a. Apple
   b. Prune
   c. Grape
   d. Orange

CHAPTER 9 · ANSWERS AND RATIONALES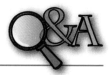

1. The answer is c.

2. The answer is b.

3. The answer is c.

4. The answer is a.

5. The answer is c.

6. The answer is d.

7. The answer is b.

8. The answer is a.

9. The answer is a.

10. The answer is d.

The toddler generally has a repeated preference for certain types of foods, refusing other types. Need for rituals related to utensils and preparation of foods persists.

Negativism is high. Rigidity, temper tantrums, self-centeredness, and a decreased attention span are normative.

Do not force the child to eat. Allow for the child's food preferences.

The best foods are bland. Introduce new foods slowly, one at a time. After age 2, lean meats and fat-modified products can be offered. Refined sweets should not be used for rewards.

Avoid toddler temper tantrums related to food. Encourage the pleasure of eating.

Growth during the toddler years is slow in terms of weight gain, but significant changes occur in body form. Muscle-mass development accounts for about half of the total weight gain. Skeletal growth decreases, but there is an increase in mineral deposition.

Six to eight teeth erupt in the beginning of the period, with the first primary teeth at 6–8 months.

Protein requirements are 13 g per day for children 1–3 years. Caloric requirements increase. The requirements for most vitamins and minerals increase slightly.

10

The Toddler (12–36 Months)

TERMS
- [ ] negativism
- [ ] finger foods
- [ ] food jags

The toddler generally has "**food jags**," or a repeated preference for certain types of foods, refusing other types. Rituals related to utensils and preparation of foods persist. Routine is very important. A typical statement of a toddler might be, "You poured the milk wrong on the cereal!"

BEHAVIORS THAT AFFECT NUTRITION

Negativism is high on the behavior list of toddlers. Rigidity, temper tantrums, self-centeredness, and a decreased attention span are normative. The toddler lacks sociability and has stranger and separation anxiety; therefore, eating in a restaurant is generally not a good idea. Physiological anorexia may be exhibited. Bowel and bladder training at this time is an added stressor, decreasing the toddler's interest in food.

WAYS TO ENHANCE NUTRITION

 Do not force the child to eat. Give the child time to get ready for meals.

Since the toddler has strong taste preferences, the best foods are bland. Offer a variety of foods from the various food groups, but allow for the child's food preferences.

Provide a routine for eating, such as allowing the child to select eating utensils. As stated previously, ritualism is important.

Serve foods attractively, do not have foods touching, and provide small portions (1 tablespoon/year of age, or one-fourth or one-third of adult portion). Introduce new foods slowly, one at a time. Give consistent, positive reinforcement to the child's attempts at new foods. Refer to foods by names that the child may find appealing, such as chicken "fingers" instead of chicken "strips."

Nutritious snacks are essential, particularly for children who do not like meals. **Finger foods** are wise choices.

Milk should be provided at the end of the meal. Two to 3 cups of milk per day allows for solid food intake. After the age of 2 years, lean meats and fat-modified products can be offered.

Do not attempt new eating behaviors when the child is tired or under stress. Meals should be as stress-free as possible. Avoid temper tantrums related to food. Give options only if there is an appropriate choice such as peanut butter or bologna. Refined sweets should not be used for rewards and should be saved for special occasions.

Food preferences are a result of direct exposure; all caregivers, even well-meaning grandparents, aunts, and uncles, should be consistent. Watch imitative behaviors that may be negative at mealtime.

Encourage the pleasure of eating. Mealtime may need to be shorter and separate from other activities. Call the child in from playing 15 minutes prior to eating. "Grazing" is okay.

NUTRITION FACTS

Growth during the toddler years is slow in terms of weight gain, but significant changes occur in body form. Muscle-mass development accounts for about half the total weight gain. Skeletal growth decreases but there is an increase in mineral deposition.

Six to eight teeth erupt in the beginning of the period. The first primary teeth at 6–8 months are the lower central incisors and then the upper central incisors. The general formula for determining the number of teeth is the age of the child in months minus 6.

Protein requirements are 13 grams/day for children 1–3 years. Caloric requirements are approximately 102 kcal/kg (about 850–1000 kcal per day) at 1 year but may increase at 2–3 years to 1400 kcal/day for the active toddler. Water requirements for this age group are 1.3 L/day. The requirements for most vitamins and minerals increase slightly during the toddler years. (Refer to Appendix A.)

2005 DIETARY GUIDELINES RECOMMENDATIONS FOR CHILDREN

- For children 2 to 3 years of age, keep total fat intake between 30 to 35% of calories, with most fats coming from sources of polyunsaturated and monosaturated fatty acids, such as fish, nuts, and vegetable oils. Always use age-appropriate foods.
- Recommended intake of potassium for children 1 to 3 years of age is 3000 mg/day from food sources.
- Children 2 to 8 years of age should consume 2 cups per day of fat-free or low-fat milk or equivalent milk products.

About Toddlers

Physical Parameters

Length
    At 2 years, average height is 34 in. (86.6 cm).
    Average growth is 3 in. (7.5 cm)/year, primarily in the legs.
    Adult height is about twice the child's height at 2 years old.
Weight
    At 2 years, average is 27 lbs.
    Average weight gain 4–6 lbs (1.8–2.7 kg)/year.
    Birth weight quadrupled by 2.5 years.

Nutritional Requirements

Calories	46 kcal/lb (102 kcal/kg)
Protein	7 g/day
Calcium	500 mg/day (DRI)
Iron	7 mg/day (DRI)
Vitamin C	15 mg/day (DRI)
Vitamin D	5 µ/day (DRI)
Folate	150 µ/day (DRI)
Zinc	3 mg/day (DRI)

Nutrition Facts

Iron	Needed for hemoglobin and blood volume
	Sources: Green leafy vegetables, legumes, grain or enriched breads, cereals, grains, dried fruits, fortified milk
Calcium	Needed for bone mineralization
	Sources: 2–3 cups of milk/day, dark green leafy vegetables, legumes
Phosphorus	Needed for bone mineralization
	Sources: Milk, eggs, meat
Vitamins	*Sources*: Fresh fruits and vegetables, fruit juices

Questions to Ask the Mother

What are the usual foods that your child eats?

Does your child engage in any food rituals or routines?

Are there any particular types of food that your child refuses?

What is a typical meal for breakfast, lunch, and dinner?

What are the types of foods that your child eats from the four basic food groups?

What utensils does your child use when eating?

What is the typical home environment during mealtime?

In what ways do you introduce new food items?

In what ways do you provide reinforcement of appropriate eating behaviors?

Has your child experienced any reactions to certain foods? If so, please describe.

CHAPTER 10 · QUESTIONS

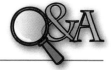

1. Chad, 2.5 years, screams when served green beans instead of canned spaghetti bits. What would you tell his caregiver?
   a. Insist that he eat the green beans and never offer the spaghetti bits.
   b. The behavior is normal for his age.
   c. Screaming is inappropriate behavior.
   d. Mix the green beans with spaghetti bits.

2. Chad does not eat when the baby-sitter serves his dinner. What is the probable cause?
   a. Rituals are important to toddlers, and he may have a routine way that he wants his dinner served.
   b. He doesn't like the baby-sitter.
   c. He wasn't hungry.
   d. He didn't like the food.

3. For preparation of Chad's food, which of the following would enhance his eating?
   a. Mix the food together.
   b. Use bland colors.
   c. Use all finger foods.
   d. Separate the foods; do not have the foods touch.

4. Which disorder is common for the toddler?
   a. Physiological anorexia
   b. Physiological jaundice
   c. Physiological bulimia
   d. Psychological anorexia

5. Chad's mother requests some suggestions for mealtime with her toddler. What would be the best suggestion for this age group?
   a. Have the child eat alone.
   b. Do not allow the child to play until he eats.
   c. Encourage the pleasure of eating; make mealtime as stress-free as possible.
   d. Do not allow "grazing."

6. One-half of the weight gain in toddlers is due to what growth activity?
   a. Skeletal growth
   b. Muscle-mass development
   c. Fat deposition
   d. Mineral deposition

7. What is the general formula for tooth development?
   a. 1 tooth each month
   b. 6–8 teeth by 3 years
   c. Central incisors appearing first at 2 years
   d. The age of the child in months minus 6

8. What are the caloric requirements for toddlers?
   a. 102 kcal/kg
   b. 300 kcal/kg
   c. 50 kcal/kg
   d. 400 kcal/kg

9. Skim or low-fat milk can be served after what age?
   a. 1 year
   b. 2 years
   c. 3 years
   d. Birth

10. What are good sources of iron for a toddler?
    a. Fruit juices and raw vegetables
    b. Milk and eggs
    c. Frozen fruits and vegetables
    d. Green leafy vegetables and enriched grains or breads

CHAPTER 10 · ANSWERS AND RATIONALES

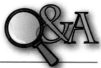

1. **The answer is b.** "Food jags" are common at this age.

2. **The answer is a.** Although the other choices may be true, rituals and routine are common dictates of the toddler's world.

3. **The answer is d.** Toddlers are more attracted to separate foods.

4. **The answer is a.** Physiological anorexia is common; toddlers are generally "picky eaters."

5. **The answer is c.** Avoid temper tantrums related to food; the less stress, the better.

6. **The answer is b.** Muscle mass is increasing.

7. **The answer is d.** This is the general rule.

8. **The answer is a.** At approximately 1 year, the requirement is 850–1000 kcal; at 3 years, 1300–1500 kcal.

9. **The answer is b.** Skim or low-fat milk should not be given until after age 2. The daily total intake of fat should be reduced to 30% of calories.

10. **The answer is d.** Of the choices, these are the best source of iron.

The preschooler's food habits are similar to those of the toddlers'. Quality is more important than quantity. Mealtime should promote positive eating behaviors.

Food fads as well as strong tastes may persist at this age. Rituals strongly influence mealtime. Finger foods are ideal. Encouraging the preschooler to self-serve is important for the development of independence.

Foods need to be prepared and served appropriately. Excessive seasoning of food should be avoided. A variety of foods and a balance of food choices promotes healthy eating.

Caloric requirements per unit of body weight continue to decrease for an upper limit of approximately 1800 kcal/day for an active child. Protein requirements rise to 19 grams/day for the 4 to 8 year old.

11

The Preschooler (3–5 Years)

TERMS
- [ ] rebellious behaviors
- [ ] finicky eaters

BEHAVIORS THAT AFFECT NUTRITION

The preschooler is challenged to develop self-feeding skills. Mealtime provides an opportunity for socialization among family members. It is important for care providers, adults, and other children to demonstrate positive eating attitudes and behaviors. The child usually initiates that behavior. It is important that a child not be forced to eat foods that are disliked.

It is important for care providers, adults, and other children to demonstrate positive eating attitudes and behaviors. The child usually imitates that behavior.

It is important that a child not be forced to eat foods that are disliked.

The preschooler's food habits are similar to those of toddlers'. Food fads as well as strong tastes may persist at this age. All preschoolers have rituals that will most likely pervade mealtime.

Preschoolers may find it difficult to sit through meals. Four-year-olds may demonstrate rebellious behaviors and have a tendency to be finicky eaters. Five-year-olds may be more agreeable to try new foods, particularly finger foods.

WAYS TO ENHANCE NUTRITION

Quality is definitely more important than quantity. But if sufficient intake is a concern, caregivers should be encouraged to keep a weekly record of a child's food intake. Foods can be measured for this record. It is important to serve small portions on small plates and use small cups. Opportunities should be provided for the child to self-regulate food intake. Finger foods are ideal; examples include raw fruits and vegetables left in a dish. Having the preschooler self-serve is imperative for the development of independence skills.

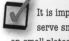

It is important to serve small portions on small plates and use small cups.

Foods need to be prepared and served appropriately; meat should be tender, crackers should be fresh, and vegetables crisp. Meals should be composed of small amounts of single foods, not combinations of foods such as stews or casseroles. Excessive seasoning of food should be avoided. Keep a variety of foods and balance food choices.

NUTRITION FACTS

Nutritional requirements for preschoolers are similar to those for toddlers (see Appendix A). Caloric requirements per unit of body weight continue to decrease, for an upper limit of approximately 1800 kcal/day for an active child.

Depending on activity level and climate total water requirements are 1.7 liters/day.

Protein requirements are 13 g/day for the 1–3-year-old, and 19 g per day for the 4–8-year-old. The caregiver needs to ensure adequate intake of calcium, fat, vitamin A, and vitamin C (e.g., fruits and vegetables).

KEY RECOMMENDATIONS OF 2005 DIETARY GUIDELINES FOR AMERICANS

- Children 2–8 years old should consume 2 cups per day of fat-free or low-fat milk or equivalent milk products.
- Keep total fat intake between 25 and 35% of calories for children and adolescents 4–18 years old with most fats coming from sources of polyunsaturated and monounsaturated fatty acids, such as nuts, fish, and vegetables.
- Intake of carbohydrates by children and adolescents needs to be monitored because increased intake of sugars may reduce fiber intake, increase calorie intake, and be a factor in the development of dental caries. Sweetened beverages and foods such as cereal are more palatable to children and adolescents, but are negatively associated with diet quality in general.
- Recommended intake of potassium for children 4–8 years old is 3800 mg/day and for 9–13-year-olds is 4500 mg/day from food sources.

Questions to Ask the Mother

What types of food does your child prefer?
What is the average length of time that your child is attentive to a task like eating?
How does your child handle new situations?
In what ways are new foods introduced?
How many people are present during meals (breakfast, lunch, dinner, snacks)?
What type of snack foods do you serve?
What type of snack foods does your child prefer?

About the Preschooler

Physical Parameters

Length
Rate of physical growth slows and stabilizes.
At 3 years, average length is 37.25 in. (95 cm).
At 4 years, average length is 40.5 in. (103 cm).
At 5 years, average length is 43.25 in. (110 cm).
Weight
At 3 years, average weight is 32 lb (14.6 kg).
At 4 years, average weight is 36.75 lb (16.7 kg).
At 5 years, average weight is 40 lb (18.1 kg).

Nutritional Requirements

Calories	1800 kcal/day–90 kcal/kg
Protein	19 g/day
Calcium	800 mg/day (DRI)
Iron	10 mg/day (DRI)
Vitamin C	25 mg/day (DRI)
Vitamin D	5 mcg/day (DRI)
Folate	200 mcg/day (DRI)
Zinc	5 mg/day (DRI)

CHAPTER 11 · QUESTIONS

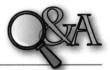

1. Jon, 4 years old, does not like mealtime; he squirms and will not sit still. What do you tell his parent?
   a. Don't worry, this is "normal" behavior for this age.
   b. He needs to be disciplined because this behavior is unacceptable.
   c. He needs to eat with other children.
   d. Go ahead and feed him.

2. Which food may be the best choice for a preschooler?
   a. Tuna noodle casserole
   b. Cream of wheat
   c. Chicken nuggets
   d. Spaghetti

3. Mary, 3 years old, has eaten only bananas for days. Her parents are very worried. What do you know about this?
   a. She is not getting enough nutrients.
   b. Food fads and strong tastes persist at this age.
   c. She must be missing an essential nutrient that bananas supply.
   d. Foods like this must be eliminated from her diet.

4. Who is most likely to try new foods?
   a. 3-year-olds
   b. 4-year-olds
   c. 5-year-olds
   d. None of the above

5. What is important to remember when assessing the nutritional status of a preschooler?
   a. Self-feeding should be encouraged.
   b. Combinations of foods are generally more likeable.
   c. Quality is more important than quantity.
   d. Seasoning makes food taste better, improving the preschooler's appetite.

6. What is one method of evaluating a preschooler's nutritional intake?
   a. Weigh the child daily.
   b. Keep a food diary.
   c. Use a slotted dish to separate foods.
   d. Use a nutritional checklist.

7. You are planning meals at a preschool. What question would be the most helpful to ask the child's caregivers?
   a. What types of snack foods does your child prefer?
   b. What time does your child usually eat?
   c. How many people are usually at meals in your home?
   d. All of the above.

8. What would also be imperative for the preschool teacher to know?
   a. Can the child sit in a chair?
   b. Can the child use a knife?
   c. How does the child feed him- or herself?
   d. How does the child handle new situations?

9. All of the following are true of the preschooler except:
   a. Nutritional requirements are similar to those for toddlers.
   b. An average of 3000 cal/day is needed.
   c. Fluid requirements decrease to 100 mL/kg/day.
   d. Protein requirements are about 24 g/day.

10. Preschoolers need an adequate amount of which combination?
   a. Calcium and fat
   b. Sugar and fat
   c. Sugar and protein
   d. Calcium and vitamin K

CHAPTER 11 · ANSWERS AND RATIONALES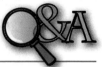

1. **The answer is a.** This behavior is very typical of the preschooler.

2. **The answer is c.** Chicken nuggets may be a good finger food choice.

3. **The answer is b.** Food fads are often prevalent for the preschooler.

4. **The answer is c.** A 5-year-old is the best bet for introducing new foods.

5. **The answer is c.** Quality is of utmost importance.

6. **The answer is b.** Maintaining a food "log" or record would help in the assessment.

7. **The answer is d.** All of these questions are appropriate.

8. **The answer is d.** Based on growth and development, the child's reaction to new situations is an important factor.

9. **The answer is b.** Requirements decrease to 90 kcal/kg for an average preschooler, for approximately 1800 cal/day.

10. **The answer is a.** Calcium and fat are needed by the preschooler to develop physically.

The school-age child may not be as hungry as the preschooler. School schedules generally dictate breakfast and lunch patterns. After-school snacking before dinner is common. The child makes independent decisions as to what he or she will eat. Weight gain may be common in preparation for puberty.

Peers influence food selection. Guidelines, especially for snacking, should be set up with the child. Exercise should be encouraged. Fat intake should be only 25–35% of the daily caloric intake.

Breakfast is the most important meal. Any food may be considered breakfast food if it is a favorite of the child's. Appropriate snacks should be provided at home and for school. A variety of fresh fruits and vegetables should be encouraged. Dental hygiene and fluoride therapy, if indicated, are musts.

Caloric requirements are 1600 kcal/day for sedentary females to 2200 kcal/day for active females, 1800 kcal/day for sedentary males to 2600 kcal/day for active males. Protein requirements for both sexes are 34 g/day or more, depending on sexual maturity. A calcium intake of 1300 kcal/day (DRI) is recommended.

Children and adolescents generally do not get enough calcium, potassium, fiber, magnesium, and vitamin E. At least half the grains consumed should be whole grains. Children 9 and older should consume 3 cups per day of fat-free or low-fat equivalent milk products; 2 cups for children 2 to 8 years. Total fat intake should be 25 to 35% of total calories for ages 4 to 18. Most fats should come from polyunsaturated

12

The School-Age Child (6–12 Years)

TERMS
- ☐ peer influence
- ☐ snacking
- ☐ sexual maturatioon

and monounsaturated fatty acids, such as nuts, fish, and vegetable oils.

Increased intake of sugars may increase caloric intake, reduce fiber intake, and contribute to dental caries.

PATTERNS OF EATING

During the school-age years, the rate of physical growth slows. Thus, the school-aged child may not be as hungry as the preschooler.

Patterns of eating may not be as flexible, as school schedules generally dictate breakfast and lunch patterns. School lunchtimes may be planned more with numbers of students in mind than when an individual is hungry. Snack time in school may be cut by the sixth grade; therefore, after-school **snacking** prior to dinner is common.

The child makes independent decisions as to what he or she will eat, not only in the school cafeteria, but also in after-school programs, or at home if caregivers are at work. Weight gain is common in preparation for puberty, which may begin as early as 9 years for girls and a few years later for boys.

> ✓ During the school-age years, the rate of physical growth slows. Thus, the school-aged child may not be as hungry as the preschooler.

BEHAVIORS THAT AFFECT NUTRITION

As the child is exposed to other dietary patterns, **peer influence** is evident in food selection. The child wants to fit in. If friends are buying lunch, the child will want to do the same. If friends bring their lunches to school, the child will want to bring what everyone else has, so as not to be ridiculed. However, caregivers should set some limits; for example, juices need to be included in the lunch bag and not soda or pop.

Guidelines, especially for snacking, should be set up with the child. Since growth slows and weight gain is common, exercise should be encouraged.

> ✓ Since growth slows and weight gain is common, exercise should be encouraged.

Overeating and obesity should not be ignored; increased weight may be carried into adulthood and may precipitate long-term adult health problems such as hypertension, diabetes, and heart disease.

Low-fat diets are not recommended, but fat intake should be only 25–35% of daily caloric intake.

WAYS TO ENHANCE NUTRITION

Breakfast is the most important meal. Studies have shown that students perform better in school when they have energy. Breakfast foods need not be traditional. As long as the

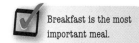
Breakfast is the most important meal.

meal is balanced, any food, including pizza or a sandwich, may be considered a "breakfast food" if it is a favorite of the child's.

Appropriate snacks should be provided at home and for school. **Snacking** on a variety of fresh fruits and vegetables should be encouraged. Crash diets should be discouraged. School-aged children may be helpful in the grocery store, where they can be given choices and asked to select nutritious foods that they enjoy.

Dental hygiene and fluoride therapy, if indicated, are musts.

NUTRITION FACTS

Caloric requirements for energy for the school-aged child range from 1600 kcal/day for sedentary females to 2200 kcal/day for active females. School-age males need 1800 kcal/day if sedentary and 2600 kcal/day if active.

Depending on **sexual maturation**, protein requirements for both sexes are 34 g/day. More lean body mass is found in children who are sexually mature; they require more protein for growth and maintenance from dietary intake. This is particularly true for boys.

Mineral and calcium requirements increase as well. For the school-ager, a calcium intake of 1300 kcal/day (DRI) is recommended. Iron and zinc are also important for growth to continue.

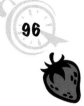

KEY RECOMMENDATIONS OF THE 2005 DIETARY GUIDELINES FOR AMERICANS

- Dietary intake data and evidence of public health problems suggest that the intake levels of calcium, potassium, fiber, magnesium, and vitamin E by children and adolescents are not sufficient.
- At least half the grains consumed by children and adolescents should be whole grains.
- Children 9 years old and older should consume 3 cups per day of fat-free or low-fat milk or equivalent milk products.
- Children 2–8 years old should consume 2 cups per day of fat-free or low-fat milk or equivalent milk products.
- Keep total fat intake between 25 and 35% of calories for children and adolescents 4–18 years old with most fats coming from polyunsaturated and monounsaturated fatty acids, such as nuts, fish, and vegetable oils.
- Intake of carbohydrates by children and adolescents needs to be monitored, because increased intake of sugars may reduce fiber intake, increase caloric intake, and be a factor in the development of dental caries. Sweetened beverages and foods such as cereal are more palatable to children and adolescents, but are negatively associated with diet quality in general.

Questions to Ask the Child

Do you eat breakfast, lunch, and dinner? With whom? Where?
What is the typical daily menu?
Do you drink milk?
Do you help with the grocery shopping?
Do you diet? How?
Do you exercise? What type?
Do you snack? What types?
Do you eat meat, poultry, and/or fish?
Do you eat when you are hungry or because everyone else is eating?
Do you throw away food from your school lunch?
Are you happy with your weight?

About the School-Age Child

Physical Parameters

Height
    Child will grow an average of 2 in. (5 cm)/year.
    Child gains 1–2 ft (30–60 cm) between ages 6 and 12.
Weight
    Child will gain 4.5–6.5 lb (2–3 kg)/year.
    Child's weight will double between ages 6 and 12.

Average 6-year-old is 45 in. (116 cm) tall and weighs 46 lb (21 kg).
Average 12-year-old is 59 in. (150 cm) tall and weighs 88 lb (40 kg).

Examples of Nutritious Snacks

Low-fat yogurt
Raisins
Fresh fruit, fruit cups
Cheese and crackers
Pretzels
Granola bars
Pudding
Fresh vegetables, such as carrots, celery
Nonsugar cereal with low-fat milk
Black pitted olives
Applesauce
Fruit juices (100%)
Low-fat milk (white and chocolate)
Whole wheat bread, English muffins
Fruit snacks

CHAPTER 12 · QUESTIONS

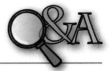

1. The mother of a 10-year-old boy is very concerned because whatever she puts in his lunch for school, he complains, "Nobody eats that!" She asks you for possible suggestions. Which of the following would be the best answer?
   a. He's just being finicky. Lay down the law.
   b. Have him buy his lunch.
   c. Give him choices for lunch. Do not select for him.
   d. Call the other childrens' parents and coordinate lunch choices.

2. Marie, 8 years old, has grown 2 inches in the past 10 months and gained 15 lb. Her family is upset by her weight gain. What is the best response you could give them?
   a. Weight gain at her age is common. Do not emphasize her weight but note if she is overeating.
   b. Do not keep any snacks in the house.
   c. Cut her caloric intake by 200 calories per day.
   d. Don't do anything; she'll slim down on her own.

3. Which of the following is the most nutritious snack?
   a. Danish and whole milk
   b. Potato chips and soda
   c. Smoothies made with fruit juice
   d. Processed cheese spread with crackers

4. Caloric intake for the school-aged child may reach which level?
   a. 1000 kcal/day
   b. 2200 kcal/day
   c. 3000 kcal/day
   d. 3500 kcal/day

5. Which is the greatest influence on the eating habits of the school-aged child?
   a. Family
   b. Siblings
   c. Teachers
   d. Peers

6. Which is the most important energy meal for the school-aged child?
   a. Breakfast
   b. Lunch
   c. Dinner
   d. Snacks

7. Fat intake for the school-aged child should be approximately:
   a. 10–20% of daily caloric intake
   b. 20–30% of daily caloric intake
   c. 25– 35% of daily caloric intake
   d. 35–50% of daily caloric intake

8. For the school-aged child, protein requirements may be as high as 46 g for what reason?
   a. Protein is needed for fat storage.
   b. As the child matures sexually, growth and maintenance require lean muscle mass.
   c. Protein causes a growth spurt.
   d. Protein prevents acne.

9. What is true of obesity in the school-aged child?
   a. It causes no harm—ignore it.
   b. It is very common and means the child is healthy.
   c. It may be detrimental later in life.
   d. It is "baby fat" that is easy to lose.

10. A boy watches television and plays videogames from after school to bedtime. You note a weight gain on his last checkup of 5 lb above normal. What do you recommend?
    a. Participation in sports
    b. Alternative activities such as bike riding
    c. Healthier after-school snacks
    d. All of the above

CHAPTER 12 · ANSWERS AND RATIONALES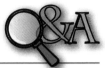

1. **The answer is c.** The child can learn to make nutritious choices with an adult's assistance.

2. **The answer is a.** Overeating or eating when she is not hungry should not be overlooked.

3. **The answer is c.** Smoothies provide a low-fat, high-vitamin snack.

4. **The answer is b.** 2200 kcal/day is generally the upper limit, depending on activity level.

5. **The answer is d.** The peer group starts to have the largest impact.

6. **The answer is a.** Energy is needed for school performance, and breakfast is the most important meal of the day.

7. **The answer is c.** Most school lunches exceed this amount.

8. **The answer is b.** Lean muscle mass is usually greater in boys.

9. **The answer is c.** The child may be more apt to develop cardiovascular disease, hypertension, and diabetes later in life.

10. **The answer is d.** All of the above are suggestions.

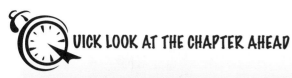

Adolescence is a period of accelerated physical growth. Eating disorders and substance abuse are ways some adolescents reduce anxiety and stress. The intake of iron, calcium, zinc, and protein should be doubled. However, the teenager usually consumes too much calories, sugar, fat, cholesterol, and sodium and not enough folic acid, vitamin B_6, and vitamin A.

Adolescence is a time of busy schedules and high stress. Meals, particularly breakfast, are often skipped. Peer relationships influence activity levels. There is increased use of carbonated beverages, caffeine, alcohol, tobacco, and recreational drugs.

The teen should have some responsibility in meal planning. Encourage healthy food choices, especially sources of calcium, iron, folate, riboflavin, and vitamins B_6, A, and C, as well as moderate exercise and group sports. Make nutritional snacks such as fresh fruits, vegetables, pretzels, popcorn, nuts, and peanut butter readily available. Discourage use of food supplements, diets, alcohol, drugs, caffeine (in coffee, tea, and carbonated drinks), nicotine, diet pills, and anabolic steroids, especially during growth spurts.

Total fat intake should be 25 to 35% of calories up to age 18, with most fats coming from nuts, fish, and vegetable oils. Girls need 2400 kcal/day if active, 1800 kcal/day if sedentary, and 46 grams of protein per day. Boys need 3200 kcal/day if active, 2200 kcal/day if sedentary, and 52 grams of protein per day. Calcium needs are 1300 mg/day for both girls and boys. Iron should be 15 mg/day for girls and 11 mg/day for boys. A pregnant teen needs the above requirements plus prenatal requirements.

13

The Adolescent (12–18 Years)

TERMS
- ☐ **sugars**
- ☐ **fats**
- ☐ **nicotine**

A high sugar level and poor hygiene encourage dental caries. Vitamins A, B, and C need to be increased. Increased levels of hormones, and not dietary habits, lead to acne. Intake levels of calcium, potassium, fiber, magnesium, and vitamin E are generally too low. At least half the grains consumed should be whole grains. The recommended intake of potassium is 4700 mg/day from food sources.

COMMON FACTORS AFFECTING NUTRITION

Adolescence is a period of accelerated physical growth. It occurs over 2 or 3 years for most individuals. Typically, there is a difference in the growth pattern between girls and boys. This period of change creates high levels of stress and anxiety for individuals. Adolescence is also a time of busy schedules and high stress. For some individuals, coping with adolescence is related to food and may lead to eating disorders. Substance abuse is another way adolescents reduce anxiety and stress.

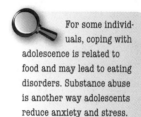

For some individuals, coping with adolescence is related to food and may lead to eating disorders. Substance abuse is another way adolescents reduce anxiety and stress.

 Both eating disorders and substance abuse severely affect adolescent nutrition.

Adolescents need adult support and role models to encourage positive methods of handling stress and anxiety.

There is a need to double the intake by adolescents of iron, calcium, zinc, and protein. The teenager takes in too much calories, sugar, fat, cholesterol, and sodium. Intake levels of certain vitamins (e.g., folic acid, vitamin B_6, and vitamin A) and minerals (iron, calcium, and zinc, in particular) are not adequate at this age.

BEHAVIORS THAT AFFECT NUTRITION

The adolescent's active lifestyle may alter food selection. With less emphasis on family meals, there is strong peer pressure to socialize while eating on the run. Frequent snacking on convenience foods and fast foods from vending machines and quick marts is common. This is the age of picky eaters, especially in girls. Meals, particularly breakfast, are often skipped.

Milk is generally replaced by carbonated beverages, and there is an increased use of caffeine, alcohol, tobacco, and recreational drugs. The adolescent is highly influenced by the media, fads, and peers. Both sexes (girls earlier than boys) are concerned with body image and are developing self-esteem and self-concept.

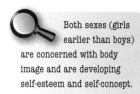

Both sexes (girls earlier than boys) are concerned with body image and are developing self-esteem and self-concept.

Adolescence is a time of many changes; the teen is searching for identity. The strongest ties are with friends. These relationships highly influence activity levels: exercise/athletics versus the couch potato.

WAYS TO ENHANCE NUTRITION

Meal plans need to be individualized, and positive feedback in response to good food choices is important. The teen should have some responsibility in meal planning. Healthy food choices, especially sources of calcium, iron, folate, riboflavin, and vitamins B_6, A, and C, should be encouraged, as well as moderate exercise and participation in group sports.

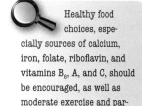

Healthy food choices, especially sources of calcium, iron, folate, riboflavin, and vitamins B_6, A, and C, should be encouraged, as well as moderate exercise and participation in group sports.

Nutritional snacks such as fresh fruits, vegetables, pretzels, popcorn, nuts, and peanut butter should be readily available. Discourage use of food supplements, diets, alcohol, drugs, caffeine (in coffee, tea, colas, and carbonated drinks), **nicotine**, diet pills, and anabolic steroids, especially during growth spurts.

NUTRITION FACTS

The 2005 Dietary Guidelines recommend a total fat intake of between 25 and 35% of calories for adolescents up to 18 years old with most fats coming from sources of polyunsaturated and monounsaturated fatty acids, such as nuts, fish, and vegetable oils.

Girls at this age generally need 2400 kcal/day if they are active, but perhaps as little as 1800 kcal/day if sedentary, and 46 g of protein per day. Boys need as much as 3200 kcal/day if active, 2200 kcal/day if sedentary, and 52 g of protein per day.

Calcium recommendations are 1300 mg/day for both girls and boys for skeletal growth and bone mineralization. Iron should be increased to 15 mg/day in girls, because of blood loss related to menstruation, and to 11 mg/day in boys because of increased blood volume and increased lean body mass due to accelerated growth.

From 10−18, the basal metabolic rate (BMR) increases, as the average boy doubles his weight and grows 13−14 in., and the average girl gains about 50 lb and grows about 9 in. The nutrition requirements of a pregnant teen include the requirements here, plus prenatal requirements. (See Chapters 2, 3, 4, and 5 for prenatal nutritional requirements.)

 The nutrition requirements of a pregnant teen include the requirements here, plus prenatal requirements. (See Chapters 2, 3, 4, and 5 for prenatal nutritional requirements.)

The high **sugar level** in the adolescent's diet and poor hygiene encourage dental caries, particularly if fluoride was not a part of the regimen in younger years.

Stress can decrease vitamin C and calcium usage; therefore, the amount of vitamins C, A, and B taken needs to be increased because deficiency is likely if the dietary intake is poor.

The B vitamins are needed to meet the demands for metabolism and growth, especially regarding muscle tissue. Increased levels of hormones such as testosterone, and not dietary habits, such as eating chocolate or potato chips, lead to acne. During the final growth spurt, body changes result from the hormonal influences that regulate the development of secondary sex characteristics.

Increased levels of hormones such as testosterone, and not dietary habits, such as eating chocolate or potato chips, lead to acne. During the final growth spurt, body changes result from the hormonal influences that regulate the development of secondary sex characteristics.

The growth rate varies widely from individual to individual, with wide fluctuations in metabolic rates and food requirements. The growth spurt is slower than in girls but boys soon will surpass the average girl in weight and height.

In girls, the amount of subcutaneous fat deposits increases, especially in the abdominal area. Hip breadth increases as the bony pelvis widens, resulting in a pelvic girdle of subcutaneous fat. In boys, there is an increase in muscle mass and long bone growth.

KEY RECOMMENDATIONS OF THE 2005 DIETARY GUIDELINES FOR AMERICANS

Based on dietary intake data and evidence of public health problems, intake levels of calcium, potassium, fiber, magnesium, and vitamin E for children and adolescents may be inadequate.

At least half the grains consumed by children and adolescents should be whole grains.

The recommended intake of potassium for adolescents is 4700 mg/day, from food sources.

Questions to Ask the Adolescent

What did you eat yesterday (24-hour dietary recall)?
Did you eat breakfast?
Did you drink milk? If so, how much and how often?
How many snacks did you have today? What kind?
When do you eat?
Where do you eat?
Do you exercise? Do you play sports? What type?
What is a typical day like for you?
Have you recently experienced any changes in your weight?
How do you feel about food and eating?
How do you relieve stress?
What do you do when you "party"?

For Girls
Have you started to menstruate?
Have your menstrual periods been regular?
How do you feel about yourself?
How do you feel when you eat?
Have you ever stopped eating?
Have you ever made yourself vomit?
Have you ever used laxatives?
Have you ever used water or diet pills?

For Boys

How do you feel about yourself?

How do you feel when you eat?

Have you ever done anything to make a certain weight class for sports
(such as not eat, take water pills, make yourself vomit, exercise ex-
cessively, perspire in a sauna, or body wrapped)?

CHAPTER 13 · QUESTIONS

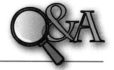

1. Who has the greatest influence on an adolescent's nutrition?
    a. Parents
    b. Peers
    c. Teachers
    d. Siblings

2. Based on the 2005 Dietary Guidelines for Americans, concern is raised regarding the lack of which nutrients in the adolescent's diet?
    a. Calcium, potassium, fiber, magnesium, and vitamin E
    b. Vitamins A and D
    c. Fats and sodium
    d. Protein and carbohydrates

3. An adolescent confides that he is having difficulty sleeping at night. Which of the following beverages would be the healthiest to drink before bedtime?
    a. Hot chocolate
    b. Soft drink
    c. Herbal tea
    d. Sport drink

4. Which statement is not true about adolescents?
    a. They are looking for their identity.
    b. Only girls are concerned about their body image.
    c. The media is major influence.
    d. They drink less milk.

5. An adolescent tells you she doesn't snack because "snack foods add unnecessary calories." What is your response?
    a. Snack foods such as raw carrots, apples, and popcorn are low in fat and calories and would supply vitamins and minerals.
    b. You are right, you should not eat between meals because your caloric need is less.
    c. It is okay to snack on diet supplement bars.
    d. Your body doesn't need any additional fat.

6. A mother tells you her adolescent son prefers to eat with his friends at a local fast-food restaurant. What suggestion might you make?
   a. Eat with him at that restaurant.
   b. Buy the food and insist he come home to eat it with his friends.
   c. Ground him.
   d. Have him be responsible for some at-home meal planning.

7. Which is an appropriate nutritional-status question to ask an adolescent?
   a. How much do you weigh?
   b. What kind of exercise do you get?
   c. Do you drink alcohol?
   d. Who do you hang out with?

8. Which question is most likely to elicit the best information from an adolescent?
   a. What is your typical day like?
   b. What did you eat for breakfast?
   c. What time did you go to sleep last night?
   d. Has your weight changed in the past 6 months?

9. Which of the following questions may best identify an adolescent girl with altered eating behaviors?
   a. With whom do you eat?
   b. Have your menstrual periods stopped?
   c. How do you feel when you eat?
   d. What foods are your favorite?

10. The adolescent tells you that she has been "very stressed out" within the past few months. What information is most important to elicit?
    a. Her grades in school
    b. Her peer group
    c. Her extracurricular activities
    d. Her possible use of alcohol or recreational drugs

11. Calcium recommendations for the adolescent are of prime importance for all of the following reasons except which one?
    a. Bone mineralization
    b. Neutralizes stomach acids
    c. Skeletal growth
    d. Prevents osteoporosis in later life

12. A total daily intake of fat for the adolescent should be how much?
    a. No more than 35% of the daily caloric intake.
    b. No more than 20% of the daily caloric intake.
    c. No fat is necessary.
    d. 45 grams per day.

CHAPTER 13 · ANSWERS AND RATIONALES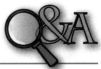

1. **The answer is b.** There is strong peer pressure at this age.

2. **The answer is a.**

3. **The answer is d.** Since the other choices all contain caffeine, a sports drink would be the most appropriate choice for insomnia.

4. **The answer is b.** Boys are also concerned with body image but usually at a later age.

5. **The answer is a.** Nutritional snacks are important to add calories and essential nutrients, particularly during growth spurts.

6. **The answer is d.** If the adolescent is responsible for planning some meals, he is more apt to participate.

7. **The answer is b.** It is important to ascertain physical activity status.

8. **The answer is a.** A typical day description is likely to elicit information about the adolescent and behaviors.

9. **The answer is c.** The adolescent may give clues to negative feelings about body image and relationships to food with answers to this question.

10. **The answer is d.** Although all are important, you need to know how the adolescent is coping with stress.

11. **The answer is b.** Calcium does not neutralize stomach acid; in fact, it may cause rebound hyperacidity.

12. **The answer is a.** Saturated fats should only comprise 10% of the total; protein intake should be at least 45 g.

Young adulthood is a high-stress period, with generally a decrease in exercise. Calcium intake is decreased, and alcohol and drugs may be misused. Smoking is on the rise, especially in women. Premenstrual syndrome may be a factor in women's eating habits. Frozen meals and fast food not nutritionally balanced may be typical choices. A balance of exercise and caloric intake is imperative. Eating small nutritious meals and snacks spread throughout the day is probably the best method to maintain weight. Dental health is a must.

For an active woman age 18–30, 2400 kcal/day is required. Women ages 31–40 require 2200 kcal/day, if active. Calcium, iron, and folate needs continue, especially for women who are considering becoming pregnant. The DRI calcium requirement is 1000 mg/day. If a woman is on oral contraceptives, lipid, blood glucose, and iron status should be monitored. Protein needs for women in this age group are 46 g/day and the iron requirement is 18 mg/day.

Intake levels of calcium, potassium, fiber, magnesium, and vitamins A (as carotenoids), C, and E, may be too low. Two cups of fruit and 2.5 cups of vegetables per day are recommended. Several times a week, consume from all five vegetable subgroups (dark green, orange, legumes, starchy vegetables, and other vegetables). Consume 3 oz or more of whole-grain products and 3 cups per day fat-free or low-fat milk or equivalent.

Women who may become pregnant should eat foods high in heme-iron and/or iron-rich plant foods or iron-fortified foods with an enhancer of iron absorption, such as vitamin C–rich foods. Women who may become pregnant and those

14

The Young Adult (18–40 Years)

TERMS
- [ ] calcium
- [ ] pregnancy
- [ ] folic acid
- [ ] whole grains

in the first trimester should consume adequate synthetic folic acid daily in addition to food forms of folate from a varied diet.

FACTORS AFFECTING NUTRITION

Young adulthood is a high-stress period. Busy schedules, earning a living, and frequent mobility come into play. During these years, young adults are developing a nuclear family of their own, or trying to find themselves if single. There is generally a decrease in exercise, and weight maintenance becomes an issue.

Foods that require little preparation are usually the norm, particularly for someone employed full-time outside the home. Calcium intake and use is decreased, and alcohol and drugs may be misused.

 Smoking is on the rise, especially by women.

Consumption of high-carbohydrate and high-fat foods by women may be evident prior to the menstrual period as a response to falling serotonin levels.

Young adult behaviors may be similar to those of adolescents, but more independent, because young adults usually have moved away from home. They are now responsible for their own nutrition and resources. They may be financially independent, but still cut corners. Meals may not be nutritionally balanced. Frozen meals and fast food may be the choices they make.

 Consumption of high-carbohydrate and high-fat foods by women may be evident prior to the menstrual period as a response to falling serotonin levels.

WAYS TO ENHANCE NUTRITION

- Young adults need to become wise shoppers, by clipping coupons, reading food labels, and comparing product ingredients and cost.
- A balance of exercise and caloric intake is imperative.
- Eating small nutritious meals and snacks spread throughout the day is probably the best method to maintain weight.
- Maintaining dental health is a must.

NUTRITION FACTS

The growth pattern of young adults is homeostatic at this point since they have reached their full genetic potential in size and strength. Typically, men have a larger muscle mass, which requires more energy and calories to maintain. For an active woman age 18–30, 2400 kcal/day is required. Women aged 31–40 require 2200 kcal/day if active. Adequate **calcium** intake (2200 to 2400 kcal/day) for active women is neccessary to maintain lean muscle mass, which is the most metabolically active tissue in the body.

Calcium, iron, and folate needs will continue, especially for women who are considering becoming pregnant. The DRI calcium requirement is 1000 mg/day to support skeletal bone mass (peak bone mass is at age 35). If a woman is on oral contraceptives, lipid, blood glucose, and iron status should be monitored.

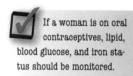

If a woman is on oral contraceptives, lipid, blood glucose, and iron status should be monitored.

During **pregnancy**, protein needs increase to 71 grams/day. The iron requirement for pregnant women is 27 mg/day. Self-imposed vegetarianism is common for this age group.

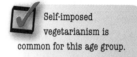

Self-imposed vegetarianism is common for this age group.

RECOMMENDATIONS OF THE 2005 DIETARY GUIDELINES FOR YOUNG ADULTS

- Maintain sufficient intake levels of calcium, potassium, fiber, magnesium, and vitamins A (as carotenoids), C, and E.
- Consume a sufficient amount of fruits and vegetables, while staying within energy needs. Two cups of fruit and 2½ cups of vegetables per day are recommended for a 2000-calorie intake, with higher or lower amounts depending on the calorie level.
- Choose a variety of fruits and vegetables each day. In particular, select from all five vegetable subgroups (dark green, orange, legumes, starchy vegetables, and other vegetables) several times per week.
- Consume 3-oz equivalents or more of whole-grain products per day, with the rest of the recommended grains coming from enriched or whole-grain products. In general, at least half the grains should be **whole grains**.

- Consume 3 cups per day of fat-free or low-fat milk or equivalent milk products.
- Women of childbearing age who may become pregnant should eat foods high in heme-iron and/or consume iron-rich plant foods or iron-fortified foods, with an enhancer of iron absorption such as vitamin C–rich foods.
- Women of childbearing age who may become pregnant and those in the first trimester of pregnancy should consume an adequate amount of synthetic folic acid daily (from fortified foods or supplements in addition to food forms of folate from a varied diet.

Questions to Ask the Young Adult

Where do you eat?

When do you eat? Throughout the day? Before bed?

What type of exercise do you get, if any?

Are you working full-time?

Are finances a concern?

Do you have medical insurance?

Do you know your family history regarding genetic problems, anemias, diabetes, etc.?

How do you feel about yourself?

Do you smoke?

Do you use drugs?

Do you drink alcohol?

Do you diet?

Do you use aids to lose weight?

Are you planning a family?

Do you feel fatigued?

Do you take vitamins?

CHAPTER 14 · QUESTIONS

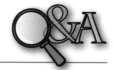

1. During young adulthood (18–40 years), which nutrient is often lacking?
   a. Iron
   b. Calcium
   c. Phosphorus
   d. Potassium

2. The nutritional status of the young adult is influenced most by which circumstance?
   a. Frequent mobility
   b. Shrinking family
   c. Less busy schedule
   d. Low stress

3. Which behavior usually occurring during young adulthood affects nutritional status?
   a. Dependence on parents
   b. Social eating patterns
   c. Premenstrual syndrome
   d. Moving away from home

4. You are taking a nutritional history from a 32-year-old. What is important to ascertain?
   a. Use of alcohol and drugs
   b. Smoking status
   c. Economic status
   d. All of the above

5. The 32-year-old tells you she is having some difficulty maintaining her weight. This is most likely due to which behavior?
   a. Eating too much
   b. Lack of exercise
   c. Homeostatic growth pattern
   d. Loss of muscle mass

6. Which is the best meal pattern for the 32-year-old to maintain her weight?
   a. Small, nutritious meals spread out throughout the day.
   b. Skip breakfast and lunch and eat a large dinner.
   c. Eat no snacks or sweetened drinks between meals.
   d. Three meals per day.

7. Which is the most metabolically active tissue in the body?
   a. Fat
   b. Bone marrow
   c. Lymph
   d. Lean muscle mass

8. Which is evidence for premenstrual syndrome as a factor in eating habits for young adult women?
   a. An increase in high-protein food due to rising serotonin levels
   b. An increase in high-carbohydrate and high-fat foods due to falling serotonin levels
   c. A decrease in high-carbohydrate and high-fat food due to falling serotonin levels
   d. A decrease in protein due to rising serotonin levels

9. Even though young adults may be financially independent, they may try to cut costs by eating what?
   a. Fresh fruits and vegetables
   b. Foods based on recipes from home
   c. Home-cooked meals
   d. Frozen and fast foods

10. A married client is using oral contraceptives. What is most important to monitor?
    a. Her weight
    b. Her height
    c. Her electrolytes
    d. Her lipid, blood glucose, and iron levels

11. Which of the following is true?
    a. Body weight decreases after age 30.
    b. Less exercise is needed as one ages.
    c. Body fat increases as one ages.
    d. Metabolism increases from 40 to 65 years.

CHAPTER 14 · ANSWERS AND RATIONALES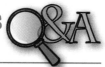

1. **The answer is b.** Calcium is often lacking due to the decrease in consumption of milk and milk products.

2. **The answer is a.** Frequent mobility is a large influence on the nutritional status of the young adult; the other choices are the opposite for this developmental period.

3. **The answer is d.** The young adult is similar developmentally to the adolescent but may be more independent.

4. **The answer is d.** All of the descriptors are important.

5. **The answer is c.** Although the other answers may also be true, most young adults gain weight because they have reached their full genetic potential in size and strength.

6. **The answer is a.** Small nutritious meals and snacks throughout the day keep a person satisfied nutritionally and prevent ravenous hunger that may lead to bingeing. If meals are eliminated, the person often makes up the calories in one large meal.

7. **The answer is d.** Muscle mass requires more energy and calories to maintain; therefore, it is more metabolically active than others.

8. **The answer is b.** Generally, consumption of high-carbohydrate and high-fat foods increases in response to falling serotonin levels.

9. **The answer is d.** Often young adults use frozen dinners and fast food to save time and money in preparation.

10. **The answer is d.** The status of lipids, blood glucose, and iron needs to be monitored because oral contraceptives may affect these levels.

11. **The answer is c.** Body fat increases after age 20 to about 35%.

Middle age is a time of body changes. Body fat content increases to 35% and lean body mass and total body water decrease to 17%. Plasma volume also decreases to 87%. Family history contributes to diseases such as type 2 diabetes mellitus, hypertension, anemia, thyroid conditions, and cancer.

Physical exercise and metabolism decrease. The rate of cell replication begins to decrease slowly. Women are at risk for osteoporosis. Exercise must be balanced with decreased caloric intake to control weight. Calcium intake needs to be maintained; if the adult is lactose-intolerant, supplements and lactose-free products may be required.

Caloric needs become less. Foods and preparation may need to be altered because of poor dentition or gastric distress. Vitamin C and vitamin B_6 may be lacking.

Women experiencing perimenopausal symptoms may crave carbohydrates and have a decreased intake of protein and calcium.

People over 50 should consume vitamin B_{12} in its crystalline form in fortified foods or supplements. Older adults, people with dark skin, and people exposed to insufficient ultraviolet radiation should consume extra vitamin D.

Individuals with hypertension, blacks, and middle-aged and older adults should consume no more than 1500 mg of sodium per day, and meet the potassium recommendation of 4700 mg/day with food.

15

The Middle-Aged Adult (40–65 Years)

TERMS
- [ ] metabolism decrease
- [ ] lifestyle modifications

FACTORS AFFECTING NUTRITION

This is a time period of body changes. Body fat content increases after age 20 to 35%, and lean body mass and total body water decrease to 17%. Plasma volume also decreases to 87%. **Metabolism decreases.** The rate of cell replication begins to decrease slowly.

Family history is important, particularly regarding the likelihood of contracting diseases such as type 2 diabetes mellitus, hypertension, anemia, thyroid conditions, or cancer.

BEHAVIORS THAT AFFECT NUTRITION

Physical exercise decreases, especially if the adult is doing sedentary work. Religious and cultural considerations influence the nutritional behavior of the middle-aged adult. Fast foods may be eaten more often if the adult works outside the home. If children are at home, the adult may finish eating their food so as not to waste it.

Women are at risk for osteoporosis, depending on their calcium intake and hormonal balance during the teen years.

WAYS TO ENHANCE NUTRITION

To control weight, exercise must be balanced with decreased caloric intake. There should be shared responsibility for buying and preparing meals if more than one person is in the household. Mealtimes should be family times and not stressful. Calcium intake needs to be maintained. If the adult is lactose intolerant (bloating, flatulence, diarrhea), calcium supplements may be needed as well as lactose-free products.

NUTRITION FACTS

Caloric needs are less in middle age, depending on lifestyle. The types of foods and preparation may need to be altered because of poor dentition or gastric distress, depending on the level of hydrochloric acid in the stomach.

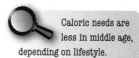

Caloric needs are less in middle age, depending on lifestyle.

The middle-aged adult may need to increase vitamin C intake, since fresh fruits and vegetables may be eaten less, owing to access and dentition state. Vitamin B_6 may also be lacking, especially if the adult consumes large amounts of alcohol.

Women experiencing perimenopausal symptoms may crave carbohydrates and take in less protein and calcium. Caffeine consumption should be decreased and intake of vitamin B_6 increased in women who have fibrocystic breast disease.

RECOMMENDATIONS OF THE 2005 DIETARY GUIDELINES FOR SPECIFIC GROUPS

- People over 50 should consume vitamin B_{12} in its crystalline form, that is, in fortified foods or supplements.
- Older adults, people with dark skin, and people exposed to insufficient ultraviolet-band radiation (i.e., sunlight) should consume extra vitamin D in vitamin D–fortified foods and/or supplements.
- Individuals with hypertension, blacks, and middle-aged and older adults should consume no more than 1500 mg of sodium per day and meet the potassium recommendation (4700 mg/day) from food.

Questions to Ask the Middle-Aged Adult

What is your method of family planning?
Where and when do you eat?
How often do you eat out?
Do you exercise formally?
What is a typical day?
How often do you see a dentist?
What is your medical history? Family history?
Do you have any metabolic problems (e.g., diabetes mellitus)?
Have you had any changes in bowel or bladder habits?
What are your habits regarding alcohol, drug use, and smoking?

For Women
Do you have any menstrual irregularities?
Do you have perimenopausal symptoms?

CHAPTER 15 · QUESTIONS

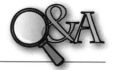

1. A 50-year-old man is concerned about gradually gaining 10 lb over the past 5 years. What should you tell him?
   a. He should not worry about it; middle-age spread is a myth.
   b. He will naturally and gradually lose the weight over the next few years.
   c. There are several products on the market he can use to reduce his weight.
   d. It may be due to a decrease in exercise that he has gained weight.

2. A mother, age 40, has 4 children under the age of 12. She states she cannot seem to lose her baby weight, even though she always plans nutritious meals that the family eats together. Which questions might you ask?
   a. Where do you shop?
   b. Do you clip coupons?
   c. Do you finish the children's food without being aware of what you're doing?
   d. How much do you spend on food?

3. The mother also tells you that as an adolescent she had difficulty with anorexia for a few years and did not menstruate. What did this put her at risk for?
   a. Osteoporosis
   b. Osteogenesis imperfecta
   c. Heart disease
   d. Early menopause

4. A man says he experiences bloating, flatulence, and diarrhea after he drinks milk. What do you expect?
   a. He is consuming too much milk.
   b. He is lactose-intolerant.
   c. He is consuming too little milk.
   d. He is sucrose-intolerant.

5. What may the man need?
   a. Calcium supplements
   b. Iron supplements
   c. Protein supplements
   d. Phosphorus supplements

6. During her last physical examination, a woman is found to have fibrocystic breasts. What dietary recommendations would you make?
   a. Do not eat spicy foods.
   b. Do not drink alcohol.
   c. Increase caffeine and decrease vitamin B_6.
   d. Decrease caffeine and increase vitamin B_6.

7. What might a perimenopausal woman crave?
   a. Protein
   b. Fats
   c. Carbohydrates
   d. Iron

8. A middle-aged adult might have difficulty consuming high-protein foods for what reason?
   a. Gastric distress
   b. Poor denition
   c. Lactose intolerance
   d. Weight constraints

9. What might be an important question to ask a middle-aged adult when assessing nutritional status?
   a. Do you have difficulty urinating?
   b. What method of family planning do you use?
   c. Do you have pain or bleeding with bowel movements?
   d. All of the above.

10. An administrative assistant (age 42) states she cannot lose weight despite decreasing her caloric intake. Which of the following recommendations is appropriate?
   a. Reduce her calories by an additional 200 cal/day
   b. Restrict her fluid intake to diet products
   c. Walk for at least 30 minutes/day
   d. Eat cold cereal for 2 meals a day

CHAPTER 15 · ANSWERS AND RATIONALES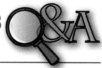

1. **The answer is d.** At this age, there may be a weight gain, especially if work is sedentary.

2. **The answer is c.** The mother may be unconsciously consuming calories by tasting and finishing foods.

3. **The answer is a.** Decreased estrogen levels can cause calcium to be drawn from bones, thereby leading to osteoporosis later in life.

4. **The answer is b.** Lactose intolerance is common in this age group.

5. **The answer is a.** Calcium supplements may be needed if the patient cannot consume milk or milk products.

6. **The answer is d.** These dietary changes may alleviate some of the discomfort associated with fibrocystic changes.

7. **The answer is c.** Carbohydrates are often the primary intake at this age.

8. **The answer is b.** Often the middle-aged adult will neglect dental health, especially if he or she does not have health insurance that covers routine cleanings.

9. **The answer is d.** All of the above are appropriate answers.

10. **The answer is C.** This follows the U.S. recommendations for healthy living.

Illness, economic status, poor dentition, inability to prepare or obtain the proper foods, social isolation, and polypharmacy may influence the ability of the older adult to eat nutritionally. Decreased eyesight, sense of smell, taste, and hearing influence appetite and enjoyment.

Physical disabilities may pose hardships in obtaining, preparing, and eating foods. Decreased renal clearance is common, and edema may occur, especially with consumption of high-sodium foods. Altered neurological states such as Alzheimer's disease may cause the individual to forget to eat.

Community and family resources can assist with obtaining and preparing food. Dental visits should be scheduled regularly. Foods should be colorful and pleasant to smell, and frequent small meals should be encouraged. Nutritional supplements may be needed. Individuals need to engage in light to moderate exercise: 30 to 60 minutes per day in addition to daily activities.

Excess supplementation is not necessary. Calcium is needed to prevent bone loss. There is a need for vitamin C. Laxatives or stool softeners may be needed. For the oldest adults (85+), physical assessment and baseline information regarding nutrition are essential.

People over 50 should consume vitamin B_{12} in its crystalline form in fortified foods or supplements. Older adults, people with dark skin, and people exposed to insufficient ultraviolet-band radiation should consume extra vitamin D from vitamin D-fortified foods and/or supplements. Individuals with hypertension, blacks, and middle-aged and

16

The Older Adult (65+ Years)

TERMS
☐ physical disabilities
☐ social isolation
☐ polypharmacy

older adults should aim to consume no more than 1500 mg of sodium per day, and meet the potassium recommendation (4700 mg/day) with food.

FACTORS AFFECTING NUTRITION

Physical, social, and economic circumstances definitely affect nutrition at the later stages of life. Poor dentition, precarious financial status, and inability to prepare or obtain food are all factors that may affect the older patient. Taking many medications can interfere with appetite and alter the metabolism and absorption of nutrients. Decreased eyesight, sense of smell, taste, and hearing also influence appetite and enjoyment of food.

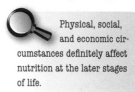

Physical, social, and economic circumstances definitely affect nutrition at the later stages of life.

Social isolation is common, particularly with the deaths of relatives and friends. Individuals may experience reduction of income due to job loss, change, or retirement.

 Weight loss can be an indicator of poor nutrition.

Physical disabilities such as arthritis may pose hardships in obtaining, preparing, and eating foods. Decreased renal clearance is common, and edema may occur, especially with consumption of high-sodium foods. Altered neurological states such as Alzheimer's disease may cause the individual to forget to eat.

The basal metabolic rate (BMR) is decreased in the older age group because of 10% less muscle mass. Physical activity and strength gradually decrease, causing decreased energy and metabolic requirements. Bone reabsorption increases with age.

BEHAVIORS THAT AFFECT NUTRITION

Elders are often "tea and toasters." Poor dentition often makes it difficult to chew foods, especially protein sources such as meats and poultry. Elders may cut corners with food if they are financially unable to buy other items such as medications. Increased devotion to religious and cultural traditions is often a mechanism for coping and for stability.

WAYS TO ENHANCE NUTRITION

Community and family resources should be secured to assist with obtaining and preparing food. Dental visits should be scheduled regularly to check the fit or need for dentures. Foods should be colorful and pleasant to smell, and frequent small meals should be encouraged. Nutritional supplements may be needed, depending on intake. Individuals need to engage in light to moderate exercise (within physical limitations) to maintain muscle mass and well-being.

NUTRITION FACTS FOR ADULTS 65–85 YEARS OLD

Excess supplementation is not necessary and may cause imbalances if other pathophysiological factors are present. Caloric requirements are decreased; however, there remains a need for calcium to prevent bone loss. Total body water, bone mass, and lean body mass decrease in the older adult. There is an overall increase in body fat mass. Therefore, weight gain is common, especially in women.

 Total body water, bone mass, and lean body mass decrease in the older adult.

There is a need for vitamin C—but not megadoses, because this may decrease the level of vitamin B_{12}. Laxatives or stool softeners may be needed, owing to decreased gastrointestinal motility.

 Mineral oil used as a laxative may reduce the absorption of fat-soluble vitamins.

Drastic changes in lifelong expectations (e.g., regarding body composition, exercise response) may produce frustration.

Based on MyPyramid, older males need only 2000 kcal/day if sedentary, and up to 2600 kcal/day if active; however, the latter number drops to 2400 kcal at age 76 years and above.

Older women require only 1600 kcal/day if sedentary, and up to 2000 kcal/day if active. These recommended caloric levels are based on the

Estimated Energy Requirements (EER) and activity levels from the Institute of Medicine Dietary Reference Intakes Macronutrients Report, 2002 (see Appendix A).

- Sedentary means less than 30 minutes per day of moderate physical activity, in addition to daily activities.
- Moderate activity is at least 30 minutes up to 60 minutes per day of moderate physical activity, in addition to daily activities.
- Active means 60 or more minutes per day of moderate physical activity, in addition to daily activities.

- Sedentary means less than 30 minutes per day of moderate physical activity, in addition to daily activities.
- Moderate activity is at least 30 minutes up to 60 minutes per day of moderate physical activity, in addition to daily activities.
- Active means 60 or more minutes per day of moderate physical activity, in addition to daily activities.

The DRI for protein is 46 g/day for both men and women. Since older individuals experience changes in body composition and decreases in lean body mass, the protein recommendation remains the same throughout adulthood to compensate for potential decreased efficiency and to maintain nitrogen balance. The DRI calcium requirement is 1200 mg/day after age 50.

Since older individuals experience changes in body composition and decreases in lean body mass, the protein recommendation remains the same throughout adulthood to compensate for potential decreased efficiency and to maintain nitrogen balance.

NUTRITION FACTS FOR OLDEST ADULTS (85+ YEARS)

After age 85, individuals experience changes in the absorption and use of nutrients. Such variations often result because of changes in gastric acid, body composition, and exercise response. It is important to obtain baseline information regarding nutrition (see Part B).

Aging results in cell breakdown. Protein synthesis can be altered due to cell damage from free radical oxidant activity. The immune and neuroendocrine systems also lose their effectiveness, resulting in decreased utilization of nutritional intake.

A continued decrease in lean body mass affects organs such as the kidneys and lungs, bone mass, and the olfactory system, resulting in a decreased sense of smell and taste.

Regular physical assessment in the elderly is essential.

Depending upon activity level and physical health, the energy requirement (kcal/day) and protein requirements for those 85 years and older are the same as for those between the ages of 65 and 85. It is essential that elderly individuals maintain a normal weight. As part of the daily intake, complex carbohydrates should be included with total carbohydrates accounting for 130 grams/day (see Appendix A). Total fiber for males should be 30 g/day and for females 21 g/day. Total water requirements for older males are 3.7 L/day and for older females 2.7 L/day.

> ✓ Depending upon activity level and physical health, the energy requirement (kcal/day) and protein requirements for those 85 years and above are the same as for those between the ages of 65 and 85.

Elderly individuals (over 70 years) need an increase of vitamin D to 15 mcg/day because of less efficient production, decreased sun exposure, and decreased activity. The eldest also benefit from vitamin B (riboflavin, pyridoxine, cobalamin).

It is very important that the elderly be assessed periodically for malnutrition, as individuals who experience decreased utilization of nutrients often will experience decreased intake, particularly of nutritious foods.

KEY RECOMMENDATIONS OF THE 2005 DIETARY GUIDELINES FOR SPECIFIC POPULATION GROUPS

- People over 50 should consume vitamin B_{12} in its crystalline form, that is, from fortified foods or supplements.
- Older adults, people with dark skin, and people exposed to insufficient ultraviolet-band radiation (i.e., sunlight) should consume extra vitamin D from vitamin D–fortified foods and/or supplements.
- Individuals with hypertension, blacks, and middle-aged and older adults should aim to consume no more than 1500 mg of sodium per day and meet the potassium recommendation (4700 mg/day) with food.

Questions to Ask the Older Adult

What, where, and how do you eat?

What is your food budget?

If in your own home:

- What is in your refrigerator?
- What is in the cupboards?

Who does your shopping and where?

Are your foods delivered?

What are your favorite foods?

Do you use canned fruits and vegetables?

What type of cooking and storage facilities do you have?

How often do you urinate?

Do you have any difficulties with urination?

How often to you defecate?

Do you have any difficulties with defecation?

What are the characteristics of your stool?

Have you experienced any unintended weight loss?

If you have dentures, do they fit properly?

About the Older Adult

Physical Assessment

Assess oral cavity for dryness and decreased salivation.

Assess for decreased sensory perceptions (taste, smell, vision), difficulty swallowing, and mental confusion.

Assess for pressure ulcers.

Assess for use of multiple medications.

Assess for recent loss, depression, and alcohol use or abuse.

Assess financial background.

Assess food-shopping practices and food preparation.

Assess for missed meals and level of snacking.

Assess for social isolation.

Assess for the presence of acute of chronic illness.

CHAPTER 16 · QUESTIONS

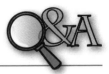

1. An older woman lives alone in a small 1-bedroom apartment. What might be one of the easiest methods to assess her nutritional status?
   a. Call her physician.
   b. Check the contents of her refrigerator.
   c. Assess her nailbeds.
   d. Ask her neighbors.

2. Why might an older adult's appetite be decreased?
   a. Diminished smell, which reduces taste
   b. Diminished hearing, which affects sensation
   c. Diminished reflexes
   d. Poor judgment

3. What does "polypharmacy" describe?
   a. Several pharmacies
   b. Several physicians
   c. Several medications
   d. A few medications

4. What exercise recommendation is appropriate for the older adult?
   a. No physical exercise because of possible injury
   b. Light to moderate exercise to maintain muscle mass and well-being
   c. Rigorous exercise to build muscles
   d. Walking only

5. What is the best meal planning for the older adult?
   a. Three meals per day and no snacks
   b. Three meals per day and one snack
   c. One large meal per day
   d. Frequent small snacks

6. Which of the following is true of the older adult?
   a. Body fat mass is increased.
   b. Body fat mass is decreased.
   c. Body fat mass is unaffected.
   d. Body composition remains unchanged from youth.

7. What does the older adult need?
   a. Calcium
   b. Vitamin C
   c. Fiber
   d. All of the above

8. A recent widower reports that he receives "meals for the elderly," yet you notice several half-eaten meal trays in his trash. What might you suspect?
   a. Depression
   b. Social isolation
   c. Both of the above
   d. None of the above

9. You are preparing a meal tray for an older man. Which of the following would be most beneficial?
   a. A bland diet
   b. A colorful meal
   c. A meal flavored with garlic
   d. Two glasses of milk

10. What is one of the most beneficial questions to ask during a nutritional history of the elderly patient?
    a. Have you experienced headaches?
    b. Have you experienced blackouts?
    c. Have you noticed a change in appetite?
    d. Have you experienced a change in appetite?

CHAPTER 16 · ANSWERS AND RATIONALES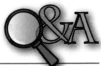

1. **The answer is b.** Checking the contents in the woman's refrigerator would tell you how much fresh food she has.

2. **The answer is a.** Smell enhances taste.

3. **The answer is c.** As a person ages, the number of prescription medications may increase for physical and mental reasons.

4. **The answer is b.** Light to moderate exercise within physical limitations is best.

5. **The answer is d.** Frequent small meals may be tolerated better.

6. **The answer is a.** Actual body fat mass is increased, although subcutaneous fat is lost.

7. **The answer is d.** All of the above are needed in increased amounts.

8. **The answer is c.** Both depression and social isolation may be contributing to his lack of appetite.

9. **The answer is b.** Color often stimulates appetite.

10. **The answer is d.** An unintended weight loss could signal illness or nutritional deficiencies.

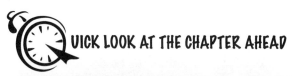

Cardiovascular disease is the number one cause of death of men and women in the United States. Cholesterol is most often associated with cardiovascular disease. Federal health officials recommend testing cholesterol levels every 5 years for adults over age 20.

There are three categories of cholesterol: very-low-density lipoprotein (VLDL), low-density lipoprotein (LDL), and high-density lipoprotein (HDL), the "good" cholesterol. Blood cholesterol assessment may therefore include lipoprotein and triglyceride levels in addition to total cholesterol level.

Genetics, sex, and age are risk factors. Others are a diet high in saturated fats, excess sugar, and excess salt; obesity; a sedentary lifestyle; smoking; and stress. Elevated homocysteine levels are a risk factor for the development of atherosclerosis. Hypertension and diabetes mellitus may be predisposing or coexisting conditions.

Dietary modifications may alleviate potential cardiovascular problems and may be used for treatment alone or in conjunction with medication. Salt, sugar, and fat all enhance flavor but add calories and cholesterol. Moderate exercise keeps weight in an acceptable range and maintains muscle mass.

Salt, sugar, and fat substitutes should be used with caution. They can cause such side effects as gastric upset, flatulence, and diarrhea. Salt substitutes generally contain potassium, so should be used cautiously by those on diuretic therapy and taking potassium supplements.

17

Cardiovascular Nutrition Therapy

TERMS
- ☐ lipids
- ☐ triglyceride
- ☐ cholesterol
- ☐ low-density lipoprotein
- ☐ high-density lipoprotein

Margarine and butter-like products may contain trans fatty acids, which may affect cholesterol and triglyceride levels.

Several dietary modifications are both palatable and therapeutic: sherbert may be substituted for ice cream, and frozen or fresh vegetables can be used instead of canned for lower sodium content. Many varieties of no-salt-added canned goods are now available.

Cardiovascular disease is the number one cause of death of men and women in the United States. Most cardiovascular disease is due to *atherosclerosis*, or the deposition of fibrous, fatty plaques along vessel walls. The progression of this narrowing of the vessels may lead to myocardial infarction, coronary heart disease, hypertension, and cerebrovascular accidents. This process begins in childhood and is affected by heredity, dietary habits, and exercise.

 Cardiovascular disease is the number one cause of death of men and women in the United States.

Several dietary factors need to be considered in the prevention and reduction of cardiovascular disease. *Hyperlipoproteinemia*, or an excess of fats in the blood, is the prime reason for the buildup of plaques. **Lipid** is the class name for fats, and **triglyceride** is the chemical name based on the chemical structure. **Cholesterol** is most often associated with cardiovascular disease; it is manufactured by the liver from saturated fats found in animal tissues.

CHOLESTEROL

Fat is not soluble in the bloodstream; it is transported by protein-wrapped molecules called *lipoproteins*, grouped according to their density or their fat and cholesterol composition into three categories:

- *very-low-density lipoprotein* (VLDL), which carries a large amount of fat to the cells and about 15% of serum cholesterol
- **low-density lipoprotein** (LDL), which transports about 60–75% of serum cholesterol from the liver to the body cells
- **high-density lipoprotein** (HDL), the "good" cholesterol, which carries 20–25% of the plasma cholesterol and collects excess cholesterol and returns it to the liver to be excreted or used to manufacture bile

Thus, blood cholesterol assessment includes more than just the total cholesterol level. It has more significance if lipoprotein levels (see Table 17-1 for values) and triglyceride levels are measured too.

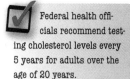

Federal health officials recommend testing cholesterol levels every 5 years for adults over the age of 20 years.

Federal health officials recommend testing cholesterol levels every 5 years for adults over the age of 20 years.

Although genetics, sex, and age are risk factors for high cholesterol that cannot be changed, other behavioral characteristics can be altered: A diet high in saturated fats, excess sugar, and excess salt; obesity; sedentary lifestyle; smoking; and stress management all play a role in the development of cardiovascular disease. Hypertension and diabetes mellitus may be predisposing or coexisting conditions. Elevated homocysteine levels recently have been implicated as a risk factor for the development of atherosclerosis.

Table 17-1 ATP III Classification of LDL, Total, and HDL Cholesterol (mg/dL)

LDL Cholesterol—Primary Target of Therapy*	
< 100	Optimal
100–129	Near optimal/above optimal
130–159	Borderline high
160–189	High
≥ 190	Very high
Total Cholesterol	
< 200	Desirable
200–239	Borderline high
≥ 240	High
HDL Cholesterol	
< 40	Low
≥ 60	High

*Determine lipoprotein levels—obtain complete lipoprotein profile after 9- to 12-hour fast.

Source: ATP III Guidelines *At-A-Glance Quick Desk Reference.* National Cholesterol Education Program. National Institutes of Health: National Heart, Lung, and Blood Institute.

CHANGING NUTRITION

From a nutritional standpoint, much can be gained for cardiovascular health by changing poor eating habits. Excess dietary sodium may cause fluid retention, which in turn raises blood pressure and increases the cardiac workload.

Caffeine will constrict blood vessels, as will smoking, increasing blood pressure and peripheral vascular resistance.

Alcohol adds excess calories, which if not burned will be deposited as fat.

Recent research shows that calcium deficiency may also lead to hypertension.

Dietary modifications alone or in conjunction with medication may be used for treatment of cardiovascular problems. Omega-3 fatty acids in fish such as cod or salmon and increasing dietary fiber are recommended to enhance cardiovascular health because the former decrease synthesis of VLDLs, and the latter lowers cholesterol.

WAYS TO ENHANCE NUTRITION

Change Dietary Habits Early

From an early age, we develop food preferences and tastes. Salt, sugar, and fat all enhance flavor but also add calories and cholesterol. Once ingrained, long-standing nutritional patterns are hard to break. Thus, it is imperative to begin teaching proper nutrition to youngsters as well as to act as good role models. Today's fast-paced, mobile society frequents fast-food "drive-thrus," not stopping long enough to see the future implications for children and adults.

Adults often claim that lower-sodium and fat-restricted meal plans are not palatable. Yet following the Food Guide Pyramid satisfies taste buds and allows for adequate amounts of nutrients and calories. Moderate exercise also keeps weight within an acceptable range and maintains muscle mass.

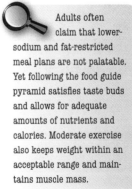

From an early age, we develop food preferences and tastes. Salt, sugar, and fat all enhance flavor but also add calories and cholesterol.

Adults often claim that lower-sodium and fat-restricted meal plans are not palatable. Yet following the food guide pyramid satisfies taste buds and allows for adequate amounts of nutrients and calories. Moderate exercise also keeps weight within an acceptable range and maintains muscle mass.

Beware Substitutes

Salt and sugar substitutes should be used sparingly. The former generally contain potassium, which should be used cautiously by those who are on diuretic therapy and taking potassium supplements.

Aspartame as a sugar substitute is not recommended in large amounts in children. Sorbitol as a sweetener may cause gastric upset and flatulence. The fat substitute olestra, used in such products as potato chips, is popular but may cause diarrhea.

A cholesterol-lowering margarine product, Benecol, whose active ingredient is a plant ester, sitostanol, is available. It inhibits transportation of cholesterol from the gastrointestinal tract to the liver. Salad dressings and spreads with the same cholesterol-lowering composition are on the market.

Long-term side effect profiles are limited for these products. Patients using it in conjunction with antihyperlipidemic medications need to be alert to negative side effects and the need for monitoring by a health care professional.

Many persons who want to lower their cholesterol levels switch to products such as margarine and lower fat butter-like products. These foods may contain trans fatty acids, which have come under scrutiny lately because researchers are unsure of how they are metabolized, and they may affect cholesterol and triglyceride levels. As of January 2006, the FDA requires food manufacturers to list trans fat content of food products on labels.

The consumer needs to read labels and be aware of what products contain.

MODIFICATIONS FOR HEALTHY LIVING

Individuals with cardiovascular disease or several risk factors can make several dietary modifications that are both palatable and therapeutic. For example, sherbert may be substituted for ice cream for lower fat. Frozen or fresh vegetables should be used instead of canned for lower sodium content. Many varieties of no-added-salt canned goods are now available. The Joint National Committee on Prevention, Detection, Evaluation and Treatment of High Blood Pressure publishes the Dietary Approaches to Stop Hypertension (DASH) Diet (see Appendix D).

Questions to Ask the Patient

What did you eat yesterday?

Who prepares your meals?

Who purchases your food?

What facilities (such as refrigerator, freezer, stove, oven, etc.) are available in your home?

How many times per week do you eat canned foods?

Do you eat frozen vegetables?

Do you eat frozen meals? What kinds?

How many meals per day do you eat and when?

Are you on a calorie-restricted or other special diet? Why? Do you follow the meal plan?

Are you taking medication (heart pill, diuretic or water pill, potassium supplements, blood pressure medicine, cholesterol-lowering medication)?

Does your income meet your needs for nutrition?

What are your food preferences? Do you like salty, sweet, fried, boiled, or baked foods?

Do your legs, feet, or hands swell? Do you have difficulty breathing, especially at night?

Do you get up to go to the bathroom during the night?

Do you have problems with constipation or diarrhea?

CHAPTER 17 · QUESTIONS

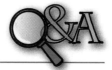

1. A woman with hypertension is taking a diuretic and a beta blocker. She tells you she knows she should not add salt to her food, but for extra flavor she uses a salt substitute. You know this may be contraindicated because:
   a. Salt substitutes cause fluid retention.
   b. Salt substitutes are expensive and don't add flavor.
   c. Salt substitutes often contain potassium and may increase potassium levels if a person is taking a diuretic and a potassium supplement.
   d. Salt substitutes often contain magnesium and may increase magnesium levels if a person is taking a diuretic and a magnesium supplement.

2. A man is concerned because his total cholesterol measures 230 mg/dL. He tells you that the "other numbers," such as VLDL, LDL, and HDL levels, do not mean anything. What would your best response be?
   a. He is correct; his cholesterol is above normal.
   b. He is correct; his cholesterol is below normal.
   c. His is not correct; the VLDL is the "good" cholesterol and should be high.
   d. He is not correct; the numbers are important and the HDL measurement is the most important.

3. A woman wants to decrease the amount of fat in her daily diet. What is the best suggestion to make?
   a. Switch from butter to margarine.
   b. Switch from whole milk to 2% fat or skim milk.
   c. Instead of eating the entire egg just eat the yolk.
   d. Eat any type of pretzel, which is lower in fat than potato chips.

4. The DASH diet may be used to prevent or stop which pathophysiological process?
   a. Hypertension
   b. Congestive heart failure
   c. Coronary artery disease
   d. Valvular disease

5. Dietary saturated fat is derived from which source?
   a. Plants
   b. Animals
   c. Vegetables
   d. All of the above

6. What makes cholesterol in the body?
   a. Gallbladder
   b. Pancreas
   c. Stomach
   d. Liver

7. The 2005 DGAs recommend what percentage of the daily caloric intake for adults be fat, particularly sources of polyunsaturated and monounsaturated fatty acids, such as fish, nuts, and vegetable oils?
   a. 10% to 25%
   b. 20% to 35%
   c. 30% to 45%
   d. 40% to 55%

8. A man, 83 years, has congestive heart failure and is being treated with digoxin and a diuretic. You review his 24-hour dietary recall and learn that he eats vegetables several times per day. What might be a valuable question?
   a. Who purchases your food?
   b. Why do you eat so many vegetables?
   c. Are the vegetables fresh, frozen, or canned, and how are they prepared?
   d. Which grocery store do you use?

9. Which of the following meat, poultry, and fish products are the lowest in saturated fats?
   a. Organ meats
   b. Duck
   c. Sausage and bacon
   d. Poultry without the skin

10. A man is concerned because his physician told him his LDL level is high. What would be your best explanation of why this might be a factor in the development of cardiovascular disease?
    a. LDL amounts are directly related to plaque formation.
    b. LDL carries cholesterol away from plaques.
    c. LDL levels really don't matter.
    d. LDL levels are only related to hypertension.

CHAPTER 17 • ANSWERS AND RATIONALES

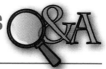

1. **The answer is c.** Additional potassium may be detrimental, particularly if the person is taking a potassium supplement. It is often hard to measure the amount of salt substitute the person is using at each meal and in cooking.

2. **The answer is d.** HDL is the "good" cholesterol and should be considered. Total cholesterol below 200 mg/dL is ideal.

3. **The answer is b.** Butter has more saturated fat but margarine still contains fat and trans fatty acids. The yolk of the egg contains the highest amount of fat, compared to the white. Some pretzels, such as honey mustard–flavored and butter-flavored, may have a high fat content as well.

4. **The answer is a.** The DASH diet was developed specifically to target lower bood pressure by dietary means.

5. **The answer is b.** Saturated fats are derived from animal sources in the diet.

6. **The answer is d.** The liver manufactures cholesterol from saturated fats.

7. **The answer is b.** This is the recommendation by both organizations.

8. **The answer is c.** Canned vegetables are high in sodium; fried vegetables will add fat.

9. **The answer is d.** All the other choices are higher in saturated fat.

10. **The answer is a.** High LDL levels increase the risk of cardiovascular disease and are directly related to the formation of plaques.

For healthy living and reducing the risk of gastrointestinal disorders, eat a balanced diet that includes grains, fresh fruits, and vegetables. Eat small, more frequent meals to facilitate digestion. Eat less fast foods; they are high in fat and sodium content. If obese, seek medical supervision for weight loss. Stop smoking. Have an annual physical examination and review of nutrition.

The gastrointestinal tract has two major functions: the mechanical and chemical breakdown of food and the absorption of digested nutrients. Partially digested food (known as **chyme**) is propelled along the intestinal tract by **peristalsis** (contraction of longitudinal muscles). Chyme in the duodenum causes the liver and gallbladder to deliver **bile** and the pancreas to deliver digestive enzymes. Bile is needed to digest and absorb fat. Absorption occurs across the intestinal wall and further metabolism occurs in the liver. The primary function of the large intestine is to absorb water and electrolytes.

Constipation is a common complaint that affects approximately 2% of the population. It is important for individuals to increase their consumption of bulk and fiber, found in whole grain cereals, raw fruits and vegetables.

Acute or chronic diarrhea can result in dehydration, electrolyte imbalance, metabolic acidosis, and weight loss. Drugs are used to suppress motility, relieve cramping and reduce stool volume and frequency. Antibiotics, diuretics, antihypertensives, and laxatives can cause diarrhea. Make sure drinking water is safe (e.g., drink bottled water) and review nutrition.

18

Digestive Disorders

TERMS
- ☐ **hormones**
- ☐ **intrinsic factors**
- ☐ **enzymes**

Gastroesophageal Reflux Disease (GERD) is the reflux of chyme from the stomach into the esophagus. Weight loss and stopping smoking can reduce the symptoms. Antacids can neutralize gastric contents. Medications can decrease acid secretions, coat ulcerated tissue, slow esophageal sphincter motility and the rate of gastric emptying.

Hiatal hernia is a protrusion of the upper part of the stomach through the diaphragm and into the thorax. Eat small, frequent meals and avoid the recumbent position after eating. Reduce weight and avoid tight-fitting clothing. Antacids reduce inflammation. Some individuals may benefit from sleeping in a semi-Fowler position.

Peptic ulcers occur when there is a disruption in the protective mucosal lining of the lower esophagus, stomach, or duodenum. Peptic ulcers can be acute or chronic, and are brought on by alcohol and nicotine use and chronic use of nonsteroidal anti-inflammatory drugs (NSAIDs).

Duodenal ulcers affect 10% to 15% of the population. Risk factors include **H. pylori** (a major cause), use of NSAIDs, and cigarette smoking. Pain is relieved rapidly by ingestion of food or antacids. Treatments include antacids, a drug to suppress acid secretion, and ulcer-coating agents such as sucralfate, colloidal bismuth, and antibiotics.

Irritable bowel syndrome symptoms range from occasional cramps and diarrhea to daily diarrhea and constipation. Fats, chocolate, alcohol, beans, and carbonated beverages make the condition worse. Treatment includes diet modification and lifestyle changes.

Crohn's disease is an inflammatory disorder. Ten to 20% of sufferers have a family history. Individuals frequently have diarrhea; pain in lower right side; weight loss; anemia; deficiencies in folic acid, vitamin D absorption, and calcium.

Diverticula are herniations of the mucosa of the colon wall. Diverticular disease occurs most commonly in the elderly. Increased dietary fiber provides symptomatic relief.

Cholelithiasis is the formation of gallstones. Cholecystitis is inflammation of the gallbladder. Cholelithiases affect 10% to 20% of the population. Treatment includes narcotics for pain control, antibiotics to manage bacterial infection, and possible surgical removal.

THE GASTROINTESTINAL TRACT

The gastrointestinal tract has two major functions: the mechanical and chemical breakdown of food and the absorption of digested nutrients. Extrinsic and intrinsic autonomic nerves and several hormones control the functions of the gastrointestinal tract. The digestive process begins in the mouth and ends with elimination.

Hormones and **enzymes** are important in the digestive process. In the stomach, *gastric* and *motilin* hormones stimulate gastric emptying, and *secretin* and *cholecystokinin* hormones delay gastric emptying. **Intrinsic factor** is secreted by gastric glands in the stomach and is needed for vitamin B_{12} absorption. The gastric glands also secrete *hydrochloric acid*, which dissolves food, kills microorganisms, and activates an enzyme called pepsin. *Maltase, sucrose*, and *lactase* are enzymes secreted by the small intestine, that help to digest proteins, carbohydrates, and fats.

DIGESTION

The digestion of food begins in the mouth where it comes into contact with *alpha amylase*, which begins carbohydrate digestion. Food is transported from the mouth to the stomach through a tube called the *esophagus*.

Once food is in the stomach, it is mixed with digestive juices and the partially digested food (known as *chyme*) is then propelled through the *pyloric valve* into the *duodenum*, which is the first part of the small intestine. The small intestine has three parts: the *duodenum,* the *jejunum,* and the *ileum.*

A process called *peristalsis* (contraction of longitudinal muscles) moves the chyme along the intestinal tract. Contraction of circular muscles (*haustral segmentation*) mixes the chyme.

The presence of chyme in the duodenum causes the liver and gallbladder to deliver *bile* and the pancreas to deliver digestive enzymes through an opening called the *sphincter of Oddi.* Bile is needed to digest and absorb fat. The liver produces it. Due to its alkaline pH, bile helps to neutralize chyme, which helps pancreatic and intestinal enzymes to digest proteins, carbohydrates, and sugars.

Absorption occurs across the intestinal wall and further metabolism occurs in the liver. Minerals and water-soluble vitamins are absorbed throughout the small intestine by active and passive transport. Sugars, amino acids, and fats are absorbed primarily in the duodenum and jejunum.

The large intestine has several parts: the *cecum, appendix, colon (ascending, transverse, descending,* and *sigmoid*), the *rectum* and the *anal canal.* The primary function of the large intestine is to absorb water and electrolytes.

There are three accessory organs of digestion: the liver, the gallbladder, and the pancreas.

The liver is the largest organ and secretes approximately 700 to 1200 mL of bile per day. The gallbladder stores the bile. When the gallbladder is stimulated by *cholecystokinin*, it contracts and secretes bile through the cystic duct and into the common bile duct. The pancreas produces two hormones called *glucagon* and *insulin,* which help with the metabolism of glucose. The pancreas also secretes several enzymes (*trypsin, chymotrypsin, carboxypeptidase, alpha amylase*, and *lipase*) that help to digest proteins, carbohydrates, and fats.

Defecation occurs when the rectum is distended with feces. There are a large number of bacteria in the colon, primarily Bacteroides, clostridia, coliforms, and lactobacilli.

COMMON CONDITIONS AND TREATMENTS

Constipation

Constipation is a common complaint that affects approximately 2% of the population. Constipation is a pattern of bowel evacuation

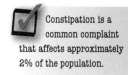
Constipation is a common complaint that affects approximately 2% of the population.

that differs among individuals and results in fewer stools, which are often hard and painful.

There are many factors that contribute to constipation. One is diet. It is important for individuals to increase their consumption of bulk and fiber found in foods such as whole-grain cereals and raw fruits and vegetables. In addition, it is important to take the time to eat, exercise, and establish a regular pattern of bowel elimination.

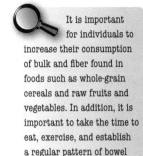 It is important for individuals to increase their consumption of bulk and fiber found in foods such as whole-grain cereals and raw fruits and vegetables. In addition, it is important to take the time to eat, exercise, and establish a regular pattern of bowel elimination.

For some individuals, depression can contribute to constipation, particularly if the individual takes anticholinergic antidepressant drugs, which inhibit motility. Other drugs, such as antacids and opiates, may also increase the risk for constipation.

Diarrhea

Diarrhea involves frequent stools and loss of fluid. Diarrhea can be acute or chronic and can result in dehydration, electrolyte imbalance, metabolic acidosis, and weight loss. It

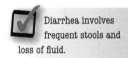 Diarrhea involves frequent stools and loss of fluid.

is important for individuals to take necessary steps to ensure that their drinking water is safe (e.g., use bottled water). Some medications such as antibiotics, diuretics, antihypertensives, and laxatives can cause diarrhea and need to be reviewed. Nutritional practices need to be evaluated and deficiencies need to be corrected. Drugs are available to suppress motility, relieve cramping, and reduce stool volume and frequency.

Gastroesophageal Reflux Disease (GERD)

GERD is the reflux of chyme from the stomach into the esophagus, due to relaxation of the lower esophageal sphincter. GERD is likely to occur 1 to 2 hours after eating. Some individuals will develop an inflammatory response known as reflux esophagitis.

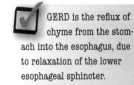 GERD is the reflux of chyme from the stomach into the esophagus, due to relaxation of the lower esophageal sphincter.

Three factors affect the severity of esophagitis: the composition of the gastric contents, the length of contact time, and the resistance of the tissue to the acid. Movement such as vomiting, coughing, lifting, or bending can increase abdominal pressure and contribute to the development of reflux esophagitis. Individuals need to evaluate their lifestyle to lessen or eliminate GERD. Weight loss and stopping smoking can reduce the symptoms. Antacids can neutralize gastric contents. Medications can decrease acid secretions, coat ulcerated tissue, and slow esophageal sphincter motility and the rate of gastric emptying.

Hiatal Hernia

Hiatal hernia is a protrusion of the upper part of the stomach through the diaphragm and into the thorax. Hiatal hernia can be exacerbated by factors that increase intra-abdominal pressure such as coughing, bending, tight clothing, ascites, or pregnancy. Since individuals with hiatal hernia often complain of reflux, dysphagia, heartburn, and epigastric pain, the presence of a myocardial infarction must be ruled out in diagnosing it. Individuals need to eat small, frequent meals and avoid the recumbent position after eating. Weight reduction is recommended. Tight-fitting clothing should be avoided. Antacids reduce the inflammation.

 Anticholinergic drugs are not used to treat hiatal hernia since they delay gastric emptying.

Some individuals may benefit from sleeping in a semi-Fowler position.

Three factors affect the severity of esophagitis: the composition of the gastric contents, the length of contact time, and the resistance of the tissue to the acid.

Individuals need to evaluate their lifestyle to lessen or eliminate GERD. Weight loss and stopping smoking can reduce the symptoms. Antacids can neutralize gastric contents. Medications can decrease acid secretions, coat ulcerated tissue, and slow esophageal sphincter motility and the rate of gastric emptying.

Hiatal hernia is a protrusion of the upper part of the stomach through the diaphragm and into the thorax.

Individuals need to eat small, frequent meals and avoid the recumbent position after eating. Weight reduction is recommended. Tight-fitting clothing should be avoided. Antacids reduce the inflammation.

Some individuals may benefit from sleeping in a semi-Fowler position.

Peptic Ulcer Disease

Peptic ulcers occur when there is a disruption in the protective mucosal lining of the lower esophagus, stomach, or duodenum. Peptic ulcers can be acute or chronic. When the mucosal lining is broken, the submucosal area is exposed to gastric secretions and autodigestion. The superficial ulcerations are called erosions since they do not penetrate the muscularis mucosae.

> Peptic ulcers occur when there is a disruption in the protective mucosal lining of the lower esophagus, stomach, or duodenum.

Blood vessel damage, hemorrhage, and possible perforation of the gastrointestinal wall can occur when the ulceration extends through the muscularis mucosae.

Lifestyle factors such as alcohol and nicotine use and chronic use of nonsteroidal anti-inflammatory drugs (NSAIDs) contribute to the development of peptic ulcer disease. Previous *Helicobacter pylori* infection is also a risk factor.

> Lifestyle factors such as alcohol and nicotine use and chronic use of nonsteroidal anti-inflammatory drugs (NSAIDs) contribute to the development of peptic ulcer disease. Previous **Helicobacter pylori** infection is also a risk factor.

Duodenal Ulcer Disease

Duodenal ulcers affect 10% to 15% of the population. Duodenal ulcers tend to occur in younger individuals, in the presence of type O blood, and affect men and women equally. The ulcers tend to recur often in the spring and fall. Complications of duodenal ulcers include intestinal obstruction, perforation, hemorrhage, hematemesis, and melena. In addition, individuals may have decreased mucosal bicarbonate secretion, hypersecretion of acid and pepsin, and rapid gastric emptying. Risk factors include *H. pylori* (a major cause), use of NSAIDs, and cigarette smoking.

> Duodenal ulcers affect 10% to 15% of the population.

Individuals with duodenal ulcers experience chronic intermittent pain in the epigastric area about 30 minutes to 2 hours after eating. The pain tends to occur in the middle of the night and disappears by morning. Pain is relieved rapidly by ingestion of food or antacids. Treatments include antacids, drugs to suppress acid secretion (e.g., cimetidine). Ulcer-coating agents such as sucralfate and colloidal bismuth and antibiotics are also useful.

Irritable Bowel Syndrome

Individuals affected by irritable bowel syndrome experience a range of symptoms from occasional cramps and diarrhea to daily pain with bowel habits of diarrhea and constipation. The exact cause is unknown. Certain foods in the diet particularly fats, chocolate, alcohol, beans, and carbonated beverages are known to make the condition worse. Treatment includes diet modification and lifestyle changes.

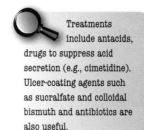
Treatments include antacids, drugs to suppress acid secretion (e.g., cimetidine). Ulcer-coating agents such as sucralfate and colloidal bismuth and antibiotics are also useful.

Crohn's Disease

Crohn's disease is an inflammatory disorder that affects both the large and small intestines. It seldom involves the rectum nor leads to the development of colon cancer. Ten to 20% of individuals have a positive family history. Immunologic factors, cigarette smoking, dietary substances, and bacteria not part of the normal flora may be contributing factors. Individuals with Crohn's disease frequently have diarrhea; pain in lower right side; weight loss; anemia; deficiencies in folic acid, vitamin D absorption, and calcium. Protein loss can lead to hypoalbuminemia. Affected individuals are at increased risk for intestinal adenocarcinoma. Treatment of Crohn's disease is usually with sulfa drugs, steroids, salicylates, and broad-spectrum antibiotics.

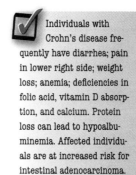
Individuals with Crohn's disease frequently have diarrhea; pain in lower right side; weight loss; anemia; deficiencies in folic acid, vitamin D absorption, and calcium. Protein loss can lead to hypoalbuminemia. Affected individuals are at increased risk for intestinal adenocarcinoma.

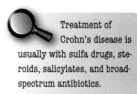
Treatment of Crohn's disease is usually with sulfa drugs, steroids, salicylates, and broad-spectrum antibiotics.

Diverticular Disease

Diverticula are herniations of the mucosa of the colon wall. Diverticular disease occurs most commonly in the elderly. The most frequent site is in the sigmoid colon. The person experiences cramping pain of the lower abdomen, diarrhea, constipation, distention, and flatulence. Inflammation can cause abscess, fever, leukocytosis, and tenderness of the lower left quadrant. Additional complications include hemorrhage, peritonitis, bowel obstruction, and fistula formation. Individuals often find increased dietary fiber provides symptom relief.

Gallbladder Dysfunction

Cholecystitis is inflammation of the gallbladder. Cholelithiasis is the formation of gallstones. Cholelithiasis affects 10% to 20% of the population. Risk factors for gallstone formation include obesity; middle age; female gender; American Indian ancestry; and gallbladder, pancreatic, or ileal disease. Frequently, individuals who have cholelithiasis experience abdominal pain, jaundice, heartburn, flatulence, epigastric discomfort, and food intolerance, especially to fats and cabbage. Gallstones can lodge in the cystic duct, which causes the gallbladder to become distended and inflamed. Pressure results in pain and decreased blood flow. Ischemia, necrosis, and perforation can occur. Most individuals will have fever, leukocytes, rebound tenderness, and abdominal muscle guarding. In diagnosis, pain must be differentiated from pancreatitis, myocardial infarction, and acute pyelonephritis of the right kidney. Treatment of gallbladder dysfunction includes narcotics for pain control, antibiotics to manage bacterial infection, and possible surgical removal.

 Cholelithiasis affects 10% to 20% of the population.

 Risk factors for gallstone formation include obesity; middle age; female gender; American Indian ancestry; and gallbladder, pancreatic, or ileal disease.

 Frequently, individuals who have cholelithiasis experience abdominal pain, jaundice, heartburn, flatulence, epigastric discomfort, and food intolerance, especially to fats and cabbage.

 Treatment of gallbladder dysfunction includes narcotics for pain control, antibiotics to manage bacterial infection, and possible surgical removal.

WAYS TO ENHANCE NUTRITION

The most important factor for healthy living and reducing risk for gastrointestinal disorders is to eat a balanced diet that includes grains, fresh fruits, and vegetables. Eating small, more frequent meals facilitates digestion. It is important to reduce the intake of fast foods due to the high amount of fat and sodium they contain. Individuals who are obese need to seek medical supervision for weight loss. Stopping smoking needs to be encouraged. Personal and familial risk factors need to be identified and effectively managed.

To prevent nutritional deficits, follow a basic, well-balanced diet. Exercise, weight management, and stress management are encouraged. Avoid foods that produce gastric distress symptoms. An annual physical examination and review of nutrition are important.

Questions to Ask the Patient

Tell me about your food intake for the past 24 hours. Is this a typical pattern for you?

Describe your consumption of bulk and fiber.

Are you currently experiencing any problems related to eating, digestion, or evacuation?

Have you ever been diagnosed with a problem related to eating, digestion, or evacuation?

Tell me about your pattern of bowel elimination. Are you concerned about any aspect?

When you have a bowel movement, have you noticed any blood or mucus?

Do you take any over-the-counter medications such as laxatives, diuretics, antacids, aspirin, or NSAIDs?

List any prescribed medications that you are currently taking (e.g., diuretics, antihypertensives, antibiotics).

Have you taken any medications for an extended period of time, now or in the past?

Are you presently or in the past have you been treated for depression? If so, for how long? Are you taking any medications for it?

What is your daily routine?

- time you get up _____
- time you go to bed _____
- what type of exercise you engage in _____
  _____
- what type of activity you are involved in (e.g., sitting, standing) while you work _____
  _____

♦ where and how you sleep _____

_____

Do you smoke cigarettes? If so, how many? _____

Do you drink alcohol? If so, how much? _____

What is your caffeine intake (e.g., coffee, soda, chocolate)? _____

_____

Is there anyone in your family who has been diagnosed with a digestive disorder (vomiting, diarrhea, constipation, GERD, hiatal hernia, peptic ulcer disease, duodenal ulcer disease, inflammatory bowel disease, Crohn's disease, diverticular disease, gallbladder dysfunction)?

MODIFICATIONS FOR HEALTHY LIVING

Suggestions for those individuals who have been diagnosed with specific digestive disorders are included in this section.

Nutritional suggestions for peptic ulcer disease:

- Currently, it is not recommended that individuals who have peptic ulcer disease follow a restrictive diet.
- Eat regular, well-balanced meals, avoid large quantities of food, decrease (eliminate) snacks, especially at bedtime.
- Avoid large quantities of milk since it stimulates gastric acid secretion, has animal fat, and lactose may increase abdominal cramping, gas, and diarrhea.
- Food seasonings are based upon individual tolerance; however, chili peppers, chili powder, and black pepper are usually not advisable.
- Use citric acid juices cautiously.
- Avoid alcohol, nicotine, caffeine, aspirin, and NSAIDs.
- Eat slowly, in a relaxed environment.

Suggestions to increase the nutrition and the integrity of the intestines for individuals who have irritable bowel syndrome:

- Ensure the intake of sufficient calories (approximately 2500 to 3000 kcal/day).
- Increase protein in the diet (approximately 100 grams/day)— suggested foods are eggs, meat, and cheese.

- Increase minerals and vitamins, especially iron, B vitamins (thiamin, riboflavin, niacin, and ascorbic acid), zinc, and potassium.
- Eat whole-grain foods, fruits, and vegetables, unless there is stenosis or individual intolerance.
- Use caution with gas-forming foods such as cabbage, brussels sprouts, broccoli, turnips, radishes, and beans.
- Reduce total fat intake.
- Eliminate/reduce caffeine, nicotine, and alcohol.
- Avoid large meals, excessive fluids (especially carbonated beverages), and gum chewing.
- Reduce eating habits that contribute to symptoms of gastric distress, e.g., avoid eating fast in a stressed environment.

Specific Questions to Ask the Patient

Have you noticed any recent changes in your eating habits?

Have you recently changed the types of foods you eat?

Have you recently noticed a change in your weight?

Do you experience any of the following symptoms: heartburn, reflux, epigastric pain?

CHAPTER 18 • QUESTIONS

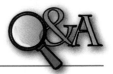

1. The gastrointestinal tract has two major functions: absorption of digested nutrients and the mechanical and _____ breakdown of food.
   a. Chemical
   b. Hormonal
   c. Autonomic
   d. Extrinsic

2. Hormones that stimulate gastric emptying are gastrin and:
   a. Secretin
   b. Motilin
   c Maltase
   d. Cholecystokinin

3. Intrinsic factor is secreted by gastric glands in the stomach and is specifically needed for the absorption of:
   a. Vitamin D
   b. Vitamin A
   c. Vitamin E
   d. Vitamin B_{12}

4. Partially digested food is known as:
   a. Plyorus
   b. Haustral
   c. Chyme
   d. Amylase

5. This digestive process moves the intestinal contents through the intestinal tract:
   a. Pylorus
   b. Haustral
   c. Peristalsis
   d. Intrinsic factor

6. The presence of chyme in the duodenum causes the liver and the gallbladder to deliver:
   a. Bile
   b. Gastrin
   c. Trypsin
   d. Chymotrypsin

7. The primary function of the large intestine is to:
   a. Digest proteins
   b. Absorb water and electrolytes
   c. Absorb vitamins and minerals
   d. Digest carbohydrates and sugars

8. Gastroesophageal reflux disease is likely to occur within what time frame after eating:
   a. 30 minutes
   b. 45 minutes
   c. 1 to 2 hours
   d. 2 to 4 hours

9. This term describes the formation of gallstones:
   a. Cholelithiasis
   b. Cholecystitis
   c. Diverticulosis
   d. Leukocytosis

10. The most frequent site of diverticulosis is:
    a. Ileum
    b. Duodenum
    c. Jejunum
    d. Sigmoid colon

CHAPTER 18 • ANSWERS

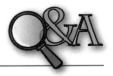

1. The answer is a.

2. The answer is b.

3. The answer is d.

4. The answer is c.

5. The answer is c.

6. The answer is a.

7. The answer is b.

8. The answer is c.

9. The answer is a.

10. The answer is d.

The kidneys make urine, act as filters for blood and body fluids, excrete the products of body metabolism, help maintain homeostasis by regulating blood pH, and regulate blood pressure. Renal disease may develop from infection, obstruction, other diseases, exposure to environmental agents, and genetic defects.

Nutritional factors must be taken into consideration when alterations occur in the kidneys. Protein consumption and sodium intake need to be monitored. Excess or retention of calcium can cause development of kidney stones.

The primary goal in the treatment of kidney disease is to maintain optimal nutritional status while simultaneously decreasing the workload of the renal system by correcting electrolyte imbalances, maintaining hydration, and reducing protein metabolism. Calcium supplements and a multivitamin may be prescribed by and taken under the guidance of a health care provider.

Careful meal planning is imperative, as essential amino acids must be ingested, while maintaining adequate protein. Consultation with a specialist or nutritionist is advisable.

Kidney stones composed of uric acid, cysteine, and struvite are unresponsive to diet modifications. Stones composed of calcium oxalate and calcium phosphate are responsive to treatment and diet modification.

19

Renal and Urinary Diet Therapy

TERMS
- ☐ **homeostasis**
- ☐ **urea**
- ☐ **creatinine clearance**

The kidneys perform several functions for the body. In addition to making urine, they act as filters for the blood and body fluids, controlling the concentration of the components and excreting the products of body metabolism.

In conjunction with the lungs, the kidneys maintain **homeostasis** by regulating blood pH.

Blood pressure is also regulated via the renin-angiotensin-aldosterone feedback mechanism and the reabsorption of fluid volume.

The functional unit of each kidney is the nephron, of which the 2,400,000 contained in the normal kidney excrete approximately 1000–1500 mL of urine each day.

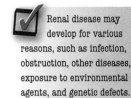
Renal disease may develop for various reasons, such as infection, obstruction, other diseases, exposure to environmental agents, and genetic defects.

Renal disease may develop for various reasons, such as infection, obstruction, other diseases, exposure to environmental agents, and genetic defects.

 Renal disease may lead to acute or chronic renal failure, possibly requiring peritoneal or hemodialysis; glomerulonephritis; nephrotic syndrome; and nephrolithiasis.

NUTRITION AND RENAL DISEASE

Since the kidneys are responsible for many excretory functions and the secretion of erythropoietin (a factor in stimulating red blood cell formation) and vitamin D (necessary to maintain the calcium-phosphorus ratio), nutritional factors must be taken into consideration when alterations occur in these organs.

Protein consumption needs to be monitored in individuals with renal conditions because an increase may overtax the failing kidney, as excess nitrogen from protein metabolism will need to be excreted, usually as **urea**.

Sodium intake also needs to be evaluated, owing to possible fluid retention and volume overload, which ultimately may lead to edema and congestive heart failure.

Excess or retention of calcium is implicated in the development of kidney stones. Dietary management plays a large role in the care of the patient with renal disease.

NUTRITIONAL TREATMENT OF KIDNEY DISEASE

Treatment of kidney disease is individualized and includes nutrition therapy. The primary goal is to maintain optimal nutritional status while simultaneously decreasing the workload of the renal system. This can be achieved by correcting electrolyte imbalances, whether due to medications or physiological processes such as vomiting and diarrhea; correcting pH; maintaining hydration; and reducing protein metabolism.

Protein is often limited to 0.5–0.6 g/kg/day or adjusted by the health care provider according to the **creatinine clearance**. If the protein level in the diet must be <20 g/day, then essential amino acid supplements can be given to retard the process of renal insufficiency.

Although fluid may be limited, it is often correlated with urine output.

Caloric intake varies according to the patient, but usually is in the range of 2000–2500 kcal/day, with about 300–400 g of carbohydrate and 75–90 g of fat to offset the lowered protein content and to provide energy. Sodium and potassium are generally restricted, the former from 500 to 2000 mg/day and the latter to about 1500 mg/day.

 As in cardiovascular disease, salt substitutes may not be appropriate owing to the potassium content of such products.

Phosphorus intake may be lowered to 500–600 mg/day, which could result in a lower calcium intake due to their combination in certain foods.

Calcium supplements and a multivitamin may be prescribed by and taken under the guidance of a health care provider.

Patients should be cautioned against buying supplements from health food stores, because the contents and effects may not be known if they are not regulated by the FDA.

MODIFICATIONS FOR HEALTHY LIVING

As discussed previously, the therapeutic renal diet may be restrictive. Processes such as osteodystrophy and loss of calcium from the bones may be unavoidable complications of long-term kidney disease. However, these pathological developments can be slowed by adherence to the prescribed restrictions.

Protein is often the prime nutritional consideration and is usually the most expensive component of the diet. Therefore, careful meal planning is imperative as essential amino acids must be ingested while protein content is adequate. Consultation with a specialist or nutritionist is often advised.

Kidney stones composed of uric acid, cysteine, and struvite are unresponsive to diet modifications. Stones composed of calcium oxalate and calcium phosphate are responsive to treatment and diet modification. (See Table 19-1.)

Table 19-1 Renal Stone Disease

Stone Chemistry	Diet Modification	Urinary pH
Calcium	low calcium (800 mg)	acid ash
Phosphate	low phosphate (1000 mg)	acid ash
Oxalate	low oxalate	acid ash

Stones composed of uric acid, cysteine, and struvite are unresponsive to diet modifications. Stones composed of calcium oxalate and calcium phosphate are responsive to treatment and diet modification.

Stanfield, P.S., & Hui, YH (2003). *Nutrition and Diet Therapy: Self-Instructional Modules.* Sudbury, MA: Jones and Bartlett Publishers, p. 341.

Questions to Ask the Patient

Do you have a meal plan? How did you develop it?

Have you seen a nutritionist?

Who purchases your food?

Who prepares your food?

What facilities are available in your home for food preparation and storage?

Is your meal plan palatable or tasty?

Do you "cheat" on your plan and if so how could it be made more to your preferences?

Do you keep a record of your intake and output?

How often do you have blood samples taken?

How often do you see your health care provider?

Do you monitor your own blood pressure?

CHAPTER 19 • QUESTIONS

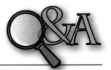

1. A man has had chronic renal failure for the past 2 years. His recent blood sample showed his creatinine clearance rate at 45 mL/minute. Based on this finding, his health care provider would most likely do which of the following to his protein consumption per day?
   a. Unrestrict it
   b. Limit it to 60 g/day
   c. Limit it to 40 g/day
   d. Limit it to 20 g/day

2. A woman has a history of calcium-based kidney stones. When taking a nutritional history, it is important for you to ask all of the following questions except which one?
   a. Do you drink milk or eat milk products, and in what amounts?
   b. Is your drinking water considered "hard"?
   c. Do you have gout?
   d. Have you been immobilized for any period of time?

3. The ability of the nephron to filter this product of protein metabolism from the blood is a measure of kidney function:
   a. Sodium
   b. Potassium
   c. Calcium
   d. BUN

4. Patients who have renal disease are often anemic because the kidneys produce the major supply of this hormone, which stimulates red blood cell production:
   a. Vitamin D
   b. Erythropoietin
   c. Antidiuretic hormone
   d. Aldosterone

5. To offset the lowered protein content of most therapeutic diets for renal disease, which of the following are generally increased to provide for energy?
   a. Carbohydrates and fats
   b. Carbohydrates and calories
   c. Calories and fat
   d. Calories alone

6. Which of the following foods contain the least amount of protein?
   a. Cheese
   b. Peanut butter
   c. Fruit
   d. Dried beans

7. If a patient is diagnosed with uric acid kidney stones, which of the following dietary modifications is most appropriate?
   a. Low phosphorus, acid ash
   b. Low calcium, acid ash
   c. Low oxalate, alkaline ash
   d. Low purine, alkaline ash

8. In acute glomerulonephritis, which of the following restrictions may not apply?
   a. Water
   b. Carbohydrates
   c. Sodium
   d. Protein

9. Which does the renin-angiotensin-aldosterone feedback mechanism help regulate?
   a. Weight
   b. Urinary output
   c. Blood pressure
   d. Appetite

10. The adequacy of protein in foods is generally categorized by its biological value. Which of the following has the least biological value protein?
    a. Meat, poultry, and fish
    b. Eggs
    c. Milk
    d. Vegetables

CHAPTER 19 · ANSWERS AND RATIONALES

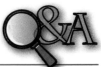

1. **The answer is a.** Usually a creatinine clearance rate of 40 mL/min and above is sufficient to metabolize unrestricted protein levels (within reason) and does not increase the progression of renal disease.

2. **The answer is c.** Gout is usually associated with uric acid stones caused by the impairment of the metabolism of purine. It is important to ascertain what types of calcium-containing foods she is eating, including milk and milk products and green leafy vegetables, and in what amounts. "Hard" water may contain more minerals including calcium. Prolonged immobilization may cause calcium to leave bones and circulate in the bloodstream.

3. **The answer is d.** BUN is an important measure of nephron and therefore kidney function.

4. **The answer is b.** In response to decreased tissue oxygenation, erythropoietin stimulates red blood cell production. When kidneys are damaged, this hormone cannot be produced in sufficient amounts.

5. **The answer is a.** Carbohydrates may be increased to 300–400 g/day and fats may be increased to 75–90 g/day.

6. **The answer is c.** Fruits contain about 0.1–1.0 g of protein per half-cup serving. The others provide about 8 g per serving.

7. **The answer is d.** Dietary restrictions of some fat and most meats will achieve a lower-purine diet. The urinary pH or dietary ash should be alkaline.

8. **The answer is b.** Carbohydrates are generally not restricted, to provide kilocalories for energy and to prevent ketosis.

9. **The answer is c.**

10. **The answer is d.** Vegetables, fruits, and cereal grains have lower biological value.

Carbohydrates are the main energy source for the body. Extra fat in the diet is not required for energy needs. Protein is generally not an energy source, but should provide 10–35% of the daily caloric intake. Generally, supplemental vitamins and minerals are not needed.

Athletic experts may recommend glycogen loading prior to competitive events involving endurance. Hydration is important for those engaged in athletic activity. For one hour or less, plain water is adequate. Longer than one hour, drinking fluids with 4–8% carbohydrate are beneficial. Glycogen stores should be replenished after intense exercise.

Adults, including older adults, need 30 minutes of moderate physical activity on nearly all days to get the most health benefits. Children and adolescents need at least 60 minutes of moderate to vigorous physical activity on most days. Pregnant women should engage in 30 minutes or more of moderately intense activity on most days.

Osteoporosis affects 25 million Americans. Fifty percent of women and 25% of men will have a fracture due to osteoporosis in their lifetime.

Modifiable behaviors associated with osteoporosis include low calcium intake, lack of weight-bearing exercise, smoking, excessive alcohol and caffeine consumption, use of medications such as corticosteroids and anticonvulsants, and coexisting medical conditions. If the amount of vitamin D is not adequate, calcium cannot be absorbed by the intestines. Persons not exposed to sunlight and

20

Musculoskeletal Diet Therapy

TERMS
☐ energy sources
☐ osteoporosis
☐ exercise

those with dark skin are at risk, including the elderly. Low levels of vitamin K have been associated with hip fractures, and some drugs, such as warfarin, may be related to bone loss. Magnesium deficiency may lead to lowered osteoclast and osteoblast activity. A high-sodium diet may also lower calcium levels.

Increase fat-free/low-fat dairy consumption to 3 cups per day; for children ages 2 to 8 years, 2 cups per day.

The Dietary Guidelines do not recommend supplements of any vitamins and minerals. All nutrients should come from food in the person's diet.

Americans have become more interested in exercising and physical fitness. Although individual programs differ, all require attention to nutrition to maintain optimal health. Often weight loss is also a goal of "working out"; thus, caloric intake may also be monitored or reduced.

ENERGY SOURCES

Carbohydrates are the main energy source for the body. Blood glucose and glycogen stored in the liver and in muscle cells provide the needed sugars. Complex carbohydrates

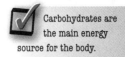
Carbohydrates are the main energy source for the body.

are considered more efficient than simple sugars since they take longer to metabolize. The AMDR for carbohydrates is 45–65% of the daily caloric intake.

Fats may be used as a fuel source from stored fatty acids in fat tissue. The AMDR of fats is 20–35% of total daily calories, with most coming from sources of polyunsaturated and monounsaturated fatty acids. This amount will supply linoleic acid, an essential amino acid.

 Extra fat in the diet is not required for energy needs.

Protein is generally not an energy source, but should provide 10–35% of the daily caloric intake. Many Americans eat more protein than they need, due to the misconception that protein builds muscle and does not lead to fat development. Excess protein strains the kidneys as they excrete the increased nitrogen, possibly leading to dehydration and increased calcium loss in the urine.

NUTRITION AND THE ATHLETE

Generally, supplemental vitamins and minerals are not needed for energy. Athletes in particular do not require increased levels of vitamins and minerals because exercise results in more efficient use of

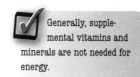

Generally, supplemental vitamins and minerals are not needed for energy.

them. Iron and folic acid deficiency may be a problem, particularly for adolescent female athletes who are menstruating and have poor dietary habits.

Hydration is important for those engaged in athletic activity. If the sporting event lasts one hour or less, plain water is adequate for hydration. If the event is longer than one hour, drinking fluids with 4–8% carbohydrate are beneficial for endurance.

Glycogen stores should be replenished after intense exercise. One to 1.5 grams of carbohydrate per kilogram of body weight (simple sugars, glucose, and sucrose) within 30 minutes after a workout, and again 2 hours later, will enhance glycogen synthesis and decrease protein breakdown. Post-exercise, 4 grams of protein for every 10 grams of carbohydrate provide additive glycogen synthesis and protein retention.

EXERCISE RECOMMENDATIONS OF THE 2005 DIETARY GUIDELINES FOR AMERICANS

- 30 minutes of moderate physical activity on nearly all days of the week provides the most health benefits for adults including reducing the risk of chronic disease.
- 60 minutes of moderate to vigorous activity on most days is needed to prevent weight gain.

- 60 to 90 minutes of moderate intensity physical activity is needed to maintain weight loss or prevent weight regain.
- The caveat to achieve the benefits of all physical activity is that the caloric intake requirements are not exceeded. A health care provider should be consulted prior to beginning a diet and exercise regimen if there are any concomitant diseases or any questions.
- Children and adolescents need at least 60 minutes of moderate to vigorous physical activity on most days for fitness, and all days of the week for healthy weight during periods of growth.
- Pregnant women should engage in 30 minutes or more of moderately intense activity on most days of the week in the absence of medical or obstetrical complications. Activities should be avoided that may cause falls or abdominal trauma.
- Breastfeeding women should be encouraged to participate in physical activity.
- Older adults should participate in physical activity as recommended, to reduce the functional declines associated with aging as well as for the health benefits.
- Recommended caloric percentage ranges to maintain BMI and long-term weight loss are carbohydrate, 45–65%; protein, 10–35%; and fat, 20–35%.

OSTEOPOROSIS

Osteoporosis, which affects 25 million Americans, is more prevalent in women (80%); however, men do develop the disease, and nearly a third has osteoporosis by age 75. Fifty percent of women and 25% of men will have a fracture due to osteoporosis in their lifetime. Osteoporosis, or literally porous bone, is a disorder of calcium metabolism. Calcium is the mineral in largest amounts in the body, primarily in bones and teeth.

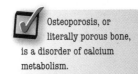
Osteoporosis, or literally porous bone, is a disorder of calcium metabolism.

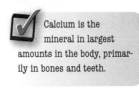
Calcium is the mineral in largest amounts in the body, primarily in bones and teeth.

Often associated with the older adult, particularly postmenopausal women, osteoporosis actually begins asymptomatically in early adulthood.

Women are more prone to osteoporosis due to nonmodifiable factors, such as heredity, smaller body frames with less bone mass, and reduced estrogen levels after menopause, which contributes to less calcium absorption and deposition.

Modifiable behaviors associated with osteoporosis include

- low calcium intake, possibly due to the misconception that dairy and calcium-rich foods are "fattening"
- lack of weight-bearing exercise
- smoking
- excessive alcohol and caffeine consumption
- use of medications such as corticosteroids and anticonvulsants
- co-existing medical conditions (rheumatoid arthritis and thyroid disease)
- conditions that may block intestinal absorption of calcium

Amenorrehic women (athletes, anorexics, bulimics) are at risk due to lack of fat to store estrogen, and men with low testosterone levels are at risk.

Calcium intake may be adequate, but interference with absorption may occur. If the amount of vitamin D is not adequate, calcium cannot be absorbed by the intestines and is excreted in urine and feces. Persons not exposed to sunlight and those with dark skin are at risk, including the elderly. Manufacturers of milk and juices are starting to fortify their products with vitamin D as well as calcium to offset responses to the health message to avoid direct sunlight and ultraviolet rays to prevent skin cancer.

Calcium absorption and excretion are also affected by alkaline, binding agents such as oxalic and phytic acids (which occur naturally in certain vegetables) and by a high-protein diet over a prolonged period of time. In light of recent popular weight-loss measures, it is thought that a high protein intake upsets the calcium/phosphorus ratio, thereby increasing calcium excretion.

When there is a low calcium level in the blood, the mineral is drawn from bones, creating low bone density (osteopenia). Ultimately, the result of chronic low calcium levels is osteoporosis.

Other vitamins and minerals are involved in the prevention of osteoporosis. Vitamin K is needed for osteocalcin synthesis. Low levels of vitamin K have been associated with hip fractures, and some drugs, such as warfarin, may be related to bone loss. Magnesium deficiency may lead to lowered osteoclast and osteoblast activity and therefore influences mineral metabolism in bone. A high-sodium diet may also lower calcium levels.

DIETARY RECOMMENDATIONS OF THE 2005 GUIDELINES FOR AMERICANS

- Increase fat-free/low-fat dairy consumption to 3 cups per day.
- For children ages 2 to 8, 2 cups of milk are recommended per day. One cup is equivalent to approximately 300 mg of calcium. Some examples of the calcium content equal to a cup of milk are 8 oz yogurt, 1½ oz cheddar cheese, 2 cups cottage cheese, 1¾ cups ice cream, 2 cups cream cheese, 2½ cups broccoli, 6 oz dry roasted almonds, 4 oz canned salmon with bones, and 15 to 24 medium-size oysters.
- The dietary guidelines do not recommend supplements of any vitamins and minerals. All nutrients should come from food in the diet unless the person is unable to eat or consume certain foods. Lactose-free milk products and/or calcium-fortified foods and beverages are suggested in that case.

MyPyramid assigns individuals to a calorie level based on their sex, age, and activity level. Table 20-1 identifies the calorie levels for males and females by age and activity level. Calorie levels are provided for each year of childhood, from 2–18 years, and for adults in 5-year increments.

Table 20-1 MyPyramid Calorie Levels

	Males				**Females**		
Activity level	**Sedentary***	**Mod. active***	**Active***	**Activity level**	**Sedentary***	**Mod. active***	**Active***
AGE				**AGE**			
2	1000	1000	1000	2	1000	1000	1000
3	1000	1400	1400	3	1000	1200	1400
4	1200	1400	1600	4	1200	1400	1400
5	1200	1400	1600	5	1200	1400	1600
6	1400	1600	1800	6	1200	1400	1600
7	1400	1600	1800	7	1200	1600	1800
8	1400	1600	2000	8	1400	1600	1800
9	1600	1800	2000	9	1400	1600	1800
10	1600	1800	2200	10	1400	1800	2000
11	1800	2000	2200	11	1600	1800	2000
12	1800	2200	2400	12	1600	2000	2200
13	2000	2200	2600	13	1600	2000	2200
14	2000	2400	2800	14	1800	2000	2400
15	2200	2600	3000	15	1800	2000	2400
16	2400	2800	3200	16	1800	2000	2400
17	2400	2800	3200	17	1800	2000	2400
18	2400	2800	3200	18	1800	2000	2400
19–20	2600	2800	3000	19–20	2000	2200	2400
21–25	2400	2800	3000	21–25	2000	2200	2400
26–30	2400	2600	3000	26–30	1800	2000	2400
31–35	2400	2600	3000	31–35	1800	2000	2200
36–40	2400	2600	2800	36–40	1800	2000	2200
41–45	2200	2600	2800	41–45	1800	2000	2200
46–50	2200	2400	2800	46–50	1800	2000	2200
51–55	2200	2400	2800	51–55	1600	1800	2200
56–60	2200	2400	2600	56–60	1600	1800	2200
61–65	2000	2400	2600	61–65	1600	1800	2000
66–70	2000	2200	2600	66–70	1600	1800	2000
71–75	2000	2200	2600	71–75	1600	1800	2000
76 and up	2000	2000	2400	76 and up	1600	1800	2000

*Calorie levels are based on the Estimated Energy Requirements (EER) and activity levels from the Institute of Medicine Dietary Reference Intakes Macro Nutrients Report, 2002.
Sedentary = up to 30 minutes a day of moderate physical activity, in addition to daily activities.
Mod. Active = 30–60 minutes a day of moderate physical activity, in addition to daily activities.
Active = 60 minutes or more a day of moderate physical activity, in addition to daily activities.

USDA Center for Nutrition Policy and Promotion, April 2005. *http://www.mypyramid.gov/professionals/pdf_calorie_levels.html*

Questions to Ask the Patient

What did you eat yesterday?

What are the frequency, intensity, and duration of your exercise on a daily or weekly basis?

Are you trying to lose weight?

What is your ideal weight?

Do you take any supplements, such as vitamins, minerals, protein, amino acids, steroids, creatine, or other body-building products?

Have you seen a health care provider recently?

What is your cardiovascular status?

How do you feel about yourself?

CHAPTER 20 · QUESTIONS

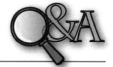

1. A man has been weight training for the past several weeks. He asks you your opinion about starting creatine supplements. What would be your best response?
   a. Ask if he has discussed this idea with his health care provider.
   b. State that the only drawback is that the supplements are very expensive.
   c. State that the supplements build a lot of muscle mass and are very good.
   d. State that the supplements are approved by the FDA.

2. A woman tells you she has been walking for 1 hour each day, 3 times per week. She also has increased her protein intake to 50% her daily caloric consumption and lowered her carbohydrate to 30% and her fat to 20%. What would be an appropriate response?
   a. That is exactly what any athlete should do to provide energy.
   b. Fat should be reduced to 10% and protein increased to 60%.
   c. The daily distribution of carbohydrates, fats, and protein need not change.
   d. Protein is the largest fuel for energy.

3. A woman wants to know if there is any danger in a high-protein diet. What should you say?
   a. Protein can be toxic to the liver.
   b. Excess protein is excreted so there is no harm.
   c. Excess protein is retained to build muscle.
   d. Excess protein taxes the kidneys because the overload of nitrogen needs to be excreted.

4. Excess protein may also cause the excretion of _____ in the urine:
   a. Phosphorus
   b. Calcium
   c. Magnesium
   d. Manganese

5. Fat intake should be approximately 25–30% of daily kilocaloric consumption in order to produce:
   a. Linoleic acid, an essential amino acid
   b. Linoleic acid, an essential trigylceride
   c. Linoleic acid, a nonessential amino acid
   d. None of the above; fat intake may be lowered

6. Which of the following activities burns the most kilocalories per hour?
   a. Weight training
   b. Modern dancing
   c. Cross-country skiing
   d. Swimming

7. A pregame meal that would enhance endurance should consist of which of the following?
   a. Pasta, bread, fruit juice
   b. Bacon, eggs, toast
   c. Waffles, sausage, coffee
   d. Steak, eggs, milk

8. What liquid provides the best hydration for an athlete?
   a. Sports drink
   b. Fruit juice
   c. Vegetable juice
   d. Water

9. What is the most common deficiency in adolescent and young adult female athletes?
   a. Calcium and phosphorus
   b. Iron and folic acid
   c. Iron and phosphorus
   d. Creatine

10. You are taking a health history from a woman and ask her about her nutritional status. Probably the best information would be obtained from her:
    a. Shopping list
    b. Food preferences
    c. 24-hour dietary recall
    d. Family

CHAPTER 20 • ANSWERS AND RATIONALES

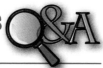

1. **The answer is a.** The body does not need the supplements since it manufactures creatine. One should talk to one's health care provider before beginning any supplements.

2. **The answer is c.** The distribution should remain the same. Proteins need only comprise 10–15% of dietary intake daily; carbohydrates and fat are the greatest energy sources.

3. **The answer is d.** The kidney acts as a filter for the by-products of protein metabolism, and excess protein can cause damage.

4. **The answer is b.** Calcium may also be excreted, leaving deficits.

5. **The answer is a.** Linoleic acid must be supplied in foods.

6. **The answer is c.** Cross-country skiing provides the most aerobic activity with the greatest caloric expenditure of these activities. Weight training exercises muscles but does not burn calories.

7. **The answer is a.** A light high-carbohydrate meal is indicated for glycogen storage.

8. **The answer is d.** Water is the best to supply hydration and satisfy thirst.

9. **The answer is b.** Iron and folic acid are often lacking due to menstruation and dietary habits.

10. **The answer is c.** The 24-hour dietary recall gives much information as to nutritional status on a daily basis.

There are four types of diabetes: type 1, type 2, gestational, and diabetes due to genetic defects in beta cell function and insulin action, diseases of the exocrine pancreas, or induced by a drug or chemical.

The classic symptoms of diabetes include polyuria, polydipsia, and unexplained weight loss. Diagnosis of diabetes includes symptoms of diabetes and a causal plasma glucose ≥ 200 mg/dL (11.1 mmol/l); or fasting plasma glucose (FPG) ≥ 126 mg/dl (7.0 mmol/l); 2-hour plasma glucose ≥200 mg/dL (11.1 mmol/L) during an oral glucose tolerance test (OGTT).

A meal plan for type 1 diabetics should be based on the individual's usual food intake, timed according to the peak action of times of insulin. Exercise under medical supervision is important.

The onset of type 2 diabetes is insidious, with nonspecific symptoms such as fatigue, pruritus, recurrent infections, visual changes, paresthesias, hyperinsulinism, and hypertension. Nutritional therapy should be directed to achieve normal glucose and lipid levels and attain normal blood pressure.

Somatic diabetic neuropathies of the lower extremities can result in difficulty in walking, muscle atrophy, and amputation. Somatic neuropathies of the upper extremities often result in sensory deficits, which can lead to such injuries as burns. Diabetic retinopathy can lead to blindness. Type 2 diabetes carries an increased risk of infections, atherosclerosis, hypertriglyceridemia,

21

Nutritional Needs of Individuals Who Have Diabetes

TERMS
- [ ] **diabetic neuropathies**
- [ ] **metabolic syndrome**

low HDL, lipoprotein oxidation, vascular consequences, altered immune mechanisms. Coronary artery diease is the most common cause of death for the type 2 diabetic.

Metabolic syndrome is associated with insulin resistance. Some people are genetically predisposed to insulin resistance and others acquire risk factors such as excess body fat, particularly central obesity, and physical inactivity.

Treatment for diabetes mellitus: maintain a desirable body weight; achieve blood glucose levels within normal parameters; have routine screenings for diabetic retinopathy and daily inspections of lower extremities for signs of adequate circulation and sensation; renal system screening of albumin, creatinine, and BUN; and monitoring of cardiovascular risk with an emphasis on plasma lipids, lipoproteins, and apolipoproteins.

Individuals who have diabetes need to decrease their intake of saturated fat and cholesterol. Obesity increases the risk for hyperlipidemia and hypertension.

Daily intake of alcohol should be limited to one drink for adult women and two drinks for adult men. Pregnant women, children, adolescents, and individuals with pancreatitis, advanced neuropathy, severe hypertriglyceridemia, or alcohol abuse should not use alcohol.

The nutritional needs of children and adolescents with diabetes are based upon healthy youth, who, in general, tend to consume too few vitamins and minerals and too much saturated fat.

Twenty percent of individuals over the age of 65 have diabetes. The same age group is at risk for polypharmacy, depression, cognitive impairment, urinary incontinence, injuries, falls, and pain.

Women already diagnosed with type 1 or type 2 diabetes will have better pregnancy outcomes if they have optimal glucose control before and during pregnancy. Women who have gestational diabetes should have adequate nutrition to maintain normal fetal weight gain, glucose levels, and absence of ketones. Consumption of carbohydrates throughout the day is very important if insulin is being used.

Hypocaloric diets (< 1200 calories per day) in obese women with gestational diabetes can result in ketonemia and ketonuria. A more modest reduction of 1600 to 1800 kcal/day results in reduced mean blood glucose levels without elevations in plasma-free fatty acids or ketonuria. Another approach to improving glucose levels is with regular aerobic exercise. Secondary benefits include cardiovascular fitness and reduced discomfort in later pregnancy.

Since breastfeeding lowers the glucose level, it is important for women with type 1, type 2, or gestational diabetes to maintain glucose levels.

Following a pregnancy affected by gestational diabetes, a woman should avoid alcoholic beverages; use nonnutritive sweeteners; distribute meals and snacks over 24 hours; make food choices to maintain normal glucose levels; attain appropriate weight gain, and absence of ketones; and engage in appropriate exercise to maintain normal glucose levels.

FOUR CLINICAL CLASSES OF DIABETES

- Type 1 diabetes resulting from beta cell destruction, and usually leading to absolute insulin deficiency
- Type 2 diabetes resulting from a progressive insulin secretory defect in addition to a history of insulin resistance
- Gestational diabetes, diagnosed during pregnancy
- Diabetes due to genetic defects in beta cell function, genetic defects in insulin action, diseases of the exocrine pancreas, and drug or chemically induced diabetes (ADA, 2005, p. 3)

CRITERIA FOR DIAGNOSIS OF DIABETES

- Symptoms of diabetes and a causal plasma glucose ≥ 200 mg/dL (11.1 mmol/L).
- Fasting plasma glucose (FPG) ≥ 126 mg/dL (7.0 mmol/L).
- Two-hour plasma glucose ≥200 mg/dL (11.1 mmol/L) during an oral glucose tolerance test (OGTT).

Causal is defined as any time of day without regard to time since last meal. Fasting is defined as no caloric intake for at least 8 hours (ADA, 2005, p. 5).

The test for diabetes should be performed as described by the World Health Organization, using a glucose load containing the equivalent of 75 g anhydrous glucose dissolved in water. It is necessary to repeat the test if positive on a different day unless there are special circumstances (ADA, 2005, p. 5). The classic symptoms of diabetes include polyuria, polydipsia, and unexplained weight loss.

The test for diabetes should be performed as described by the World Health Organization, using a glucose load containing the equivalent of 75 g anhydrous glucose dissolved in water. It is necessary to repeat the test if positive on a different day unless there are special circumstances (ADA, 2005, p. 5).

TYPE 1 DIABETES

Type 1 diabetes mellitus affects the metabolism of fat, protein, and carbohydrates. As glucose accumulates in the blood, the renal

The classic symptoms of diabetes include polyuria, polydipsia, and unexplained weight loss.

threshold for glucose is exceeded, and glucose appears in the blood. The individual experiences the symptoms of polyuria and thirst as a result of changes in osmotic diuresis. The lack of insulin causes protein and fat to be broken down, which results in weight loss. The individual who has type 1 diabetes mellitus experiences polydipsia, polyuria, polyphagia, weight loss, and hyperglycemia in fasting and postprandial states.

Individuals with type 1 diabetes must ensure sufficient calories to achieve and maintain normal weight for height and age. It is necessary to base dietary needs upon age, activity, and severity of the diabetes. It is important to develop a meal plan based on the individual's usual food intake, so that meals and snacks can be planned according to the peak action times of insulin.

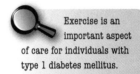 It is important to develop a meal plan based on the individual's usual food intake, so that meals and snacks can be planned according to the peak action times of insulin.

Exercise is an important aspect of care for individuals with type 1 diabetes mellitus. Exercise must be under medical supervision, since it can result in serious outcomes such as hypoglycemia, hyperglycemia, ketosis, cardiovascular ischemia, dysrhythmia, exacerbation of proliferative retinopathy, and lower extremity injury.

Exercise is an important aspect of care for individuals with type 1 diabetes mellitus.

TYPE 2 DIABETES

Individuals who have type 2 diabetes mellitus experience cellular resistance to the effect of insulin. There is a high incidence of type 2 among individuals who are Native Americans, Hispanic/Latino American, and African American. Additional risk factors include inactivity, illnesses, medications, age (over 40), and obesity.

The onset of type 2 diabetes is insidious. Individuals often experience nonspecific symptoms such as fatigue, pruritus, recurrent infections, visual changes, paresthesias, hyperinsulinism, and hypertension.

It is important for individuals with type 2 diabetes to follow a medically supervised weight-loss program, since this often results in improved glucose tolerance.

Nutritional therapy should be goal directed to achieve normal glucose and lipid levels and attain normal blood pressure. Exercise is an important aspect of treatment since it can not only result in weight loss, but it also reduces postprandial blood glucose levels, lowers triglycerides and cholesterol levels, and increases HDL cholesterol.

Some individuals may also require oral medications that primarily affect glucose tolerance/resistance. Effective medications such as sulfonylureas, biguanid metformin, thiazolidinediones, and alpha-glucosidase inhibitor acarbose are important aspects of therapy. Insulin therapy may also be necessary at times for individuals who have type 2 diabetes mellitus (ADA, 2005, p. 9).

CONDITIONS RELATED TO DIABETES

Diabetic neuropathies result from the interaction of multiple metabolic, genetic, and environmental factors. Underlying pathology includes a combination of vascular and metabolic factors that can result in diabetic neuropathies.

Somatic neuropathies of the lower extremities can result in difficulty in walking, muscle atrophy, and amputation. Somatic neuropathies of the upper extremities often result in safety issues related to sensory deficits such as burns. Diabetic retinopathy produces visual changes and can lead to eventual blindness.

Individuals with type 2 diabetes are also at increased risk for infections, atherosclerosis, hypertriglyceridemia, low HDL, lipoprotein oxidation, vascular consequences, and altered immune mechanisms. Coronary artery disease is the most common cause of death in individuals with type 2 diabetes.

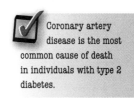

Coronary artery disease is the most common cause of death in individuals with type 2 diabetes.

Metabolic syndrome is a collection of risk factors experienced by one person, associated with a generalized metabolic disorder called insulin resistance (also called insulin resistance syndrome). Symptoms include central obesity, atherogenic dyslipidemia (mainly high triglycerides and low HDL cholesterol), raised blood pressure, insulin resistance or glucose intolerance, pro-thrombolic state (high fibrinogen or plasminogen activator inhibitor), and pro-inflammatory state (elevated high-sensitivity C-reactive protein in the blood).

Some people are genetically predisposed to insulin resistance and other individuals acquire risk factors such as excess body fat, particularly central obesity, from physical inactivity.

The diagnostic criteria for metabolic syndrome includes three or more of the following: central obesity as measured by waist circumference (men > 40 inches, women > 35 inches); fasting blood triglycerides ≥ 150 mg/dL; blood HDL cholesterol (men < 40 mg/dL, women < 50 mg/dL); blood pressure ≥ 130/85 mm Hg; fasting glucose ≥ 110 mg/dL (American Heart Association, 2005).

KEY RECOMMENDATIONS FOR NUTRITION

The focus of treatment for individuals who have diabetes mellitus is a nutritional intake that meets basic metabolic needs for development and maintenance of the body.

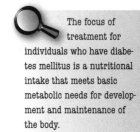

The focus of treatment for individuals who have diabetes mellitus is a nutritional intake that meets basic metabolic needs for development and maintenance of the body.

- It is essential that an appropriate diet for diabetes mellitus be developed and followed to achieve and maintain a desirable body weight.
- Another aspect of treatment is to achieve blood glucose levels that are within the normal parameters.
- It is also important to prevent complications through routine screenings, such as annual screening for diabetic retinopathy and daily inspections of lower extremities for signs of adequate circulation and sensation.
- Since diabetes also affects the renal system, routine screening of albumin, creatinine, and BUN are important.
- Reduction of cardiovascular risk is essential and needs to be monitored with an emphasis on plasma lipids, lipoproteins, and apolipoproteins.

Individuals who have diabetes mellitus require a treatment program that is centered on adequate nutrition. The diet is based on the nutritional needs of that individual for normal growth and development, physical activity, and maintenance of a desirable lean weight. It is important in devising a diet for diabetes mellitus to consider the total requirements of kilocalories for energy; the percentage of kilocalories allotted to carbohydrates, protein, and fat; and a general food distribution pattern for the day.

According to the Food and Agriculture Organization of the United Nations and the World Health Organization, the preferred terms for food carbohydrates are sugars, starch, and fiber. The previously used terms (simple sugars, complex carbohydrates, and fast-acting carbohydrates) are poorly defined and should no longer be used (ADA, 2005).

 It is important in devising a diet for diabetes mellitus to consider the total requirements of kilocalories for energy, the percentage of kilocalories allotted to carbohydrates, protein, and fat; and a general food distribution pattern for the day.

Carbohydrates

There is strong evidence to support the need for carbohydrates taken in from whole grains, fruits, vegetables, and low-fat milk in the diet. However, with regard to the glycemic effects of carbohydrates, the total amount of carbohydrate in meals and snacks is more important than the source or type. The percentage of carbohydrates should be based on an individual nutrition assessment. Carbohydrate and monounsaturated fat together should provide 60% to 70% of energy intake for individuals with type 1 or 2 diabetes. Individuals receiving intensive insulin therapy should adjust their premeal insulin dosages based on the carbohydrate content of meals.

 Individuals receiving intensive insulin therapy should adjust their premeal insulin dosages based on the carbohydrate content of meals.

The use of low-glycemic-index food may reduce postprandial hyperglycemia, but there is not sufficient evidence of long-term benefit to recommend use of low-glycemic-index diets as a primary strategy in food/meal planning for individuals with type 1 diabetes. Consumption of fiber is to be encouraged; however, there is no reason to recommend that people with type 1 diabetes consume a greater amount of fiber than other individuals. A consistent carbohydrate intake is recommended for individuals receiving a fixed daily insulin dosage (Franz et al., 2002, p. 8).

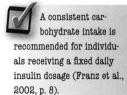 *A consistent carbohydrate intake is recommended for individuals receiving a fixed daily insulin dosage (Franz et al., 2002, p. 8).*

Sugars

There has been an assumption that nutrition planning for individuals with diabetes should include restriction of added natural and added sugars, since both contributed to hyperglycemia. However, what needs to take place is planning. If sucrose is going to be consumed, then it needs to be substituted for other carbohydrates and/or covered with adequate insulin or glucose-lowering medication (Franz et al., 2002, p. 11).

Protein

Protein intake for individuals with type 1 or type 2 diabetes averages 15% to 20% of total energy intake. Ingested protein does not increase plasma glucose concentrations in individuals with controlled type 2 diabetes; however, ingested protein will serve as a potent stimulant of insulin secretion, similar to carbohydrates.

There is no evidence to suggest that the usual protein intake should be decreased if renal function is normal. The effect of high protein intake (> 20% of total energy) on the development of nephropathy has not been determined.

What is known at this point indicates that dietary protein does not slow the absorption of carbohydrates, and dietary protein and carbohydrate do not raise plasma glucose later than carbohydrate alone and thus do not prevent late-onset hypoglycemia.

It is unknown what long-term effects a diet high in protein and low in carbohydrate will have on individuals with diabetes and on plasma LDL cholesterol (Franz et al., 2002, p. 17).

Fat

In order to decrease plasma LDL cholesterol and the risk of coronary heart disease, energy derived from saturated fat should be reduced. This can be achieved if saturated fat is replaced with carbohydrates if weight loss is desirable, or with monounsaturated fat if weight loss is not a goal. It is suggested that polyunsaturated fat intake be ~10% of energy intake. Ethnic and cultural backgrounds need

It is suggested that polyunsaturated fat intake be ~10% of energy intake.

Ethnic and cultural backgrounds need to be considered when planning low-fat diets.

to be considered when planning low-fat diets. Individuals may use low-fat food and fat replacers/substitutes to help reduce total fat and energy intake and thereby facilitate weight loss (Franz et al., 2002, p. 21).

Obesity

Individuals who have type 2 diabetes often become obese (~36% have a BMI $\geq$ 30.0 kg/m^2). Obesity increases insulin resistance and the risk for hyperlipidemia and hypertension. Weight reduction is therefore a focus of the therapeutic treatment program for type 2 diabetes.

Lifestyle changes include eating a balanced diet that provides daily vitamin and mineral requirements from natural food sources, taking an appropriate multivitamin (avoiding mega-dosing), education, regular physical exercise, and behavior modification (Franz et al., 2002, p. 26).

Alcohol

If an individual chooses to drink alcohol, daily intake should be limited to one drink for adult women and two drinks for adult men. One drink is defined as a 12-oz beer, or a 5-oz glass of wine, or a 1.5-oz glass of distilled spirit. Blood glucose levels are not affected when moderate amounts of alcohol are consumed. Alcohol should be consumed with food to reduce the risk of hypoglycemia.

 Excessive, chronic ingestion of alcohol will raise a person's blood pressure and possibly increase the risk for a stroke.

Pregnant women, children, adolescents, and individuals who have medical problems such as pancreatitis, advanced neuropathy, severe hypertriglyceridemia, or alcohol abuse should not drink alcohol (Franz et al., 2002, p. 32).

CONSIDERATIONS FOR SPECIFIC POPULATION GROUPS

Children and Adolescents

Achieving appropriate and relatively stable blood glucose levels without excessive episodes of hypoglycemia is the focus of care for children and adolescents who have type 1 diabetes. The best approach to this goal is with individualized food and meal planning, flexible insulin regimens and algorithms, self-blood glucose monitoring, education, and promoting decision making based on outcomes. For youth who have type 2 diabetes, the focus of care is on the promotion of healthy lifestyle and treatment goals to normalize glucose levels (Franz et al., 2002, p. 36).

Very little research has been published on the nutritional needs of children and adolescents who have diabetes; therefore, the recommendations are based upon healthy youth—who tend to be deficient in vitamins and minerals and above the recommended levels of saturated fat. Children and adolescents who have type 1 diabetes usually experience weight loss and will require insulin management, hydration, and adequate energy intake.

The best strategy for managing children with type 1 diabetes is a food/nutrition history based upon a 1- to 3-day food record of meals evaluated in terms of weight gain and growth, based upon the pediatric growth chart from the Centers for Disease Control. This evaluation should be completed every 3 to 6 months, depending upon progress (Franz et al., 2002, p. 36).

Children and adolescents need to be screened initially for and monitored periodically for lipid abnormalities. Their total fat, saturated fat, and cholesterol levels need to be within the levels in current published guidelines. It is recommended that children over 2 years of age increase their dietary fiber to an amount equal to or greater than their age plus 5 g/day (Franz et al., 2002, p. 36).

For youth with type 2 diabetes, the focus of treatment is nutrition therapy and exercise to achieve the goals of preventing excessive weight gain, achieving appropriate

> The best strategy for managing children with type 1 diabetes is a food/nutrition history based upon a 1- to 3-day food record of meals evaluated in terms of weight gain and growth, based upon the pediatric growth chart from the Centers for Disease Control. This evaluation should be completed every 3 to 6 months, depending upon progress (Franz et al., 2002, p. 36).

> For youth with type 2 diabetes, the focus of treatment is nutrition therapy and exercise to achieve the goals of preventing excessive weight gain, achieving appropriate linear growth, establishing stable blood glucose levels and stable HbA1c. Nutrition therapy needs to address hypertension and dyslipidemia by teaching strategies to decrease intake of high-caloric, high-fat foods and to encourage exercise.

linear growth, establishing stable blood glucose levels and stable HbA1c. Nutrition therapy needs to address hypertension and dyslipidemia by teaching strategies to decrease intake of high-caloric, high-fat foods and to encourage exercise.

Older Individuals

At least 20% of individuals over the age of 65 have diabetes. In addition, this same age group is also at risk for polypharmacy, depression, cognitive impairment, urinary incontinence, injuries, falls, and pain.

An involuntary change in body weight, a loss or gain greater than 10 pounds or 10% of body weight in less than 6 months, needs to be evaluated to determine if it is nutritionally related (Franz et al., 2002, p. 42). The energy requirement for older adults is 20% to 30% less than a younger adult. It is important to remember that a too-low body weight is associated with greater morbidity and mortality in the older adult.

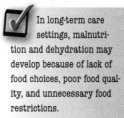

The energy requirement for older adults is 20% to 30% less than a younger adult.

In long-term care settings, malnutrition and dehydration may develop because of lack of food choices, poor food quality, and unnecessary food restrictions. It is necessary to consider alternatives in food planning that may involve changing meds rather than food restrictions in order to enhance nutrition and achieve glucose level control.

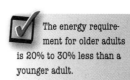

In long-term care settings, malnutrition and dehydration may develop because of lack of food choices, poor food quality, and unnecessary food restrictions.

Dietary fiber is important to the total plan, as well as hydration (Franz et al., 2002, p. 42). Specific vitamins and minerals to evaluate closely include vitamin C, vitamin D, vitamin B_{12}, thiamine, calcium, zinc, and magnesium. (See Appendix A for DRIs.)

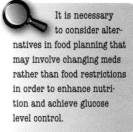

It is necessary to consider alternatives in food planning that may involve changing meds rather than food restrictions in order to enhance nutrition and achieve glucose level control.

Pregnant Women

Women already diagnosed with type 1 or type 2 diabetes will have better pregnancy outcomes if they have optimal glucose control before and during pregnancy.

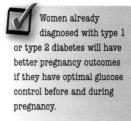

Women already diagnosed with type 1 or type 2 diabetes will have better pregnancy outcomes if they have optimal glucose control before and during pregnancy.

It is important for women with diabetes to recognize the relationship between their food plan, eating habits (eating regularly, including an evening snack), glucose levels, and the expected physiological effects of pregnancy on the body (Franz et al., 2002, p. 39).

The treatment goal for women who have gestational diabetes is to promote adequate nutrition to maintain the maternal and fetal health necessary for appropriate fetal weight gain, normal glucose levels, and the absence of ketones. Meals and snacks should be spread across the day to ensure appropriate glucose levels without accelerated ketosis overnight. A diet with 40% to 45% of total energy intake from carbohydrates is effective is reducing postprandial glucose levels.

> The treatment goal for women who have gestational diabetes is to promote adequate nutrition to maintain the maternal and fetal health necessary for appropriate fetal weight gain, normal glucose levels, and the absence of ketones.

Carbohydrates are not tolerated as well at breakfast for most women; however, it is important to evaluate glucose response to food at different times during the day. Consistency in use of carbohydrates throughout the day is very important if insulin is added to the care of the woman (Franz et al., 2002, p. 40).

The use of hypocaloric diets (< 1200 calories per day) in obese women with gestational diabetes can result in ketonemia and ketonuria. A more modest reduction of 1600 to 1800 kcal/day results in reduced mean blood glucose levels without elevations in plasma-free fatty acids or ketonuria. It is important that daily food records, weekly weight checks, and ketone testing be used to determine individual energy recommendations for the obese gestational diabetic.

> It is important that daily food records, weekly weight checks, and ketone testing be used to determine individual energy recommendations for the obese gestational diabetic.

Another approach to improving glucose levels is with regular aerobic exercise. Secondary benefits include cardiovascular fitness and reduced discomfort in later pregnancy. At least three exercise sessions per week of 15 minutes over 2 to 4 weeks is necessary to modify glucose levels (Franz et al., 2002, p. 40).

Women need to recognize their risk for developing gestational diabetes in a subsequent

> Women need to recognize their risk for developing gestational diabetes in a subsequent pregnancy and for developing type 2 diabetes later in life. There needs to be a discussion of lifestyle behavior changes for weight reduction and increased physical activity in order to reduce subsequent risk of diabetes.

pregnancy and for developing type 2 diabetes later in life. There needs to be a discussion of lifestyle behavior changes for weight reduction and increased physical activity in order to reduce subsequent risk of diabetes.

BREASTFEEDING

A woman with type 1 or type 2 diabetes or gestational diabetes may choose to breastfeed. Since breastfeeding lowers the glucose level, it is important for a breastfeeding woman to maintain her glucose levels. If a woman uses insulin, it may be necessary for her to eat snacks with carbohydrates either before or after breakfast, along with an evening or late-night snack.

Some diabetic women may require an increase of ~200 calories above the usual pregnancy meal plan during the first six months of breastfeeding. Most women can tolerate an 1800-kcal/day diet.

KEY RECOMMENDATIONS

- Reduce weight and increase physical activity following a pregnancy affected by gestational diabetes.
- Avoid use of alcoholic beverages.
- Use nonnutritive sweeteners.
- Distribute meals and snacks over a 24-hour time period.
- Choose foods to maintain normal glucose levels, attain appropriate weight gain, and avoid ketones.
- Exercise to maintain normal glucose levels.
- Breastfeeding is possible with appropriate meal planning.

Questions to Ask the Diabetic

Tell me about your symptoms related to diabetes mellitus.

How long have you experienced symptoms related to diabetes mellitus?

In what ways do you deal with your feelings regarding diabetes mellitus?

What foods have you eaten in the past 24 hours? Is this typical?

What is your typical pattern of daily activity?

What types of exercise do you engage in?
Are you currently taking insulin? If so, how much?
Are you currently taking an oral hypoglycemic agent? If so, which one?
Do you currently see a dietitian?
Have you noticed a recent change (loss or gain) in your weight?
What type of fats (saturated/unsaturated) are in your diet?
Do you drink alcohol? If yes, describe the amount and type.
Do you monitor your blood sugar? If yes, by what method?
Do you take vitamin supplements?
Do you take any herbs?
Do you do your own shopping?
Do you do your own cooking?
Do you follow planning principles for food preparation?
Do you need to review (learn) meal planning principles?

SUGGESTIONS TO IMPROVE NUTRITIONAL INTAKE

- Use less meat and more grains.
- Purchase lean cuts of meat.
- Cut off all visible fat prior to cooking.
- Eat 2–3-ounce portions (cooked).
- Remove the skin.
- Use low-fat milk.

MODIFICATIONS FOR HEALTHY LIVING

- Establish a working relationship with a team of health care providers (physician, nurse, and nutritionist).
- Engage in preventive care, such as routine screenings and thorough physical exams.
- Establish blood glucose levels within normal limits and ideal weight by following a recommended diet plan.
- Establish a medically supervised exercise plan.
- Keep a log of reactions to diet, activity, and use of insulin or oral hypoglycemic agents in order to have accurate information for care providers as they monitor your care plan.

SOURCES

American Diabetes Association. (2005). Standards of medical care in diabetes. *Diabetes Care, (S1), 28,* 4–36.

Franz, M., Bantle, J., Beebe, C., Chiasson, J., Barg, A., Holzmeister, L., Hoogwerf, B., Mayer-Davis, E., Mooradian, A., Purnell, J., Wheeler, M. (2002). Evidence-based nutrition principles and recommendations for the treatment and prevention of diabetes and related complications. *Diabetes Care, 25,* 148–198.

CHAPTER 21 · QUESTIONS

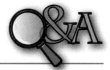

1. This type of diabetes results from beta cell destruction and usually leads to absolute insulin deficiency:
   a. Type 1
   b. Type 2
   c. Gestational diabetes
   d. Impaired glucose tolerance

2. The diagnosis of diabetes is based on which of the following lab values related to fasting plasma glucose level:
   a. 80 mg/dL
   b. 100 mg/dL
   c. 126 mg/dL
   d. 200 mg/dL

3. For adults who are diagnosed with diabetes, what percentage of the total calories should be derived from carbohydrate and monounsaturated fats:
   a. 15% to 20%
   b. 25% to 50%
   c. 55% to 60%
   d. 60% to 70%

4. This type of diabetes results from an insulin secretory defect that is progressive in addition to a history of insulin resistance:
   a. Type 1
   b. Type 2
   c. Gestational diabetes
   d. Combination diabetes

5. For individuals older than 65 years of age with diabetes, an involuntary change in body weight, loss or gain greater than _____ pounds or _____ of body weight in less than 6 months needs to be evaluated to determine if it is nutritionally related.
   a. 5 pounds/5%
   b. 10 pounds/10%
   c. 15 pounds/15%
   d. 20 pounds/20%

6. Metabolic syndrome is recognized as a collection of risk factors that include insulin resistance, central obesity, elevated triglycerides, and high blood pressure. Part of the diagnostic criteria includes an elevated fasting blood glucose level above:
   a. 110 mg/dL
   b. 120 mg/dL
   c. 130 mg/dL
   d. 140 mg/dL

7. The classic symptoms of diabetes include polyuria, polydipsia, and:
   a. Gastritis
   b. Nausea
   c. Fatigue
   d. Weight loss

8. Protein intake for individuals with type 1 or type 2 diabetes averages _____ of adult energy intake.
   a. 5% to 10%
   b. 15% to 20%
   c. 25% to 30%
   d. 35% to 40%

9. It is recommended that children over 2 years of age increase their dietary fiber to an amount equal to or greater than their age plus:
   a. 2 grams/day
   b. 5 grams/day
   c. 8 grams/day
   d. 10 grams/day

10. It is suggested the level of polyunsaturated fat intake for individuals who have diabetes mellitus be:
    a. ~10% of energy intake
    b. ~20% of energy intake
    c. ~30% of energy intake
    d. ~40% of energy intake

CHAPTER 21 • ANSWERS AND RATIONALES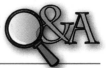

1. The answer is a.

2. The answer is c.

3. The answer is d.

4. The answer is b.

5. The answer is b.

6. The answer is a.

7. The answer is d.

8. The answer is b.

9. The answer is b.

10. The answer is a.

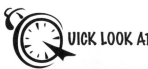

Cancer is an abnormality in cell structure or function. Nutrition plays an integral role in the development of and recovery from cancer. It is important to complete a personal nutrition assessment to identify the individual's needs (based on type, location, and extent of the cancer), current nutritional status, and personal desires, tolerances, and dislikes.

If an adult has good nutrition, a daily diet of about 2000 kcal is sufficient. However, if the adult is malnourished, the calorie requirement may be as high as 3000–4000 kcal.

It is important to have adequate carbohydrate intake to prevent further tissue destruction. Ideally, carbohydrates should supply the majority of calories, and fat should account for approximately 30% or less of the intake.

Protein intake may need to be increased to meet maintenance needs and prevent protein wasting.

Adequate vitamins and minerals are essential in the treatment of individuals who have cancer.

Sufficient fluid intake is necessary. Fluids help to eliminate the breakdown products of chemotherapy agents and destroyed cancer cells. In addition, adequate fluid intake protects the urinary tract from irritation and inflammation.

22

Nutritional Needs of Cancer Patients

TERMS
- ☐ sarcomas
- ☐ carcinomas

FACTORS AFFECTING NUTRITION

Cancer results when there is an abnormality in cell structure or function as a result of out-of-control cell reproduction. Cancer tumor types are classified by the source of the involved tissue: **Sarcomas** originate from connective tissue and **carcinomas** arise from epithelial tissue. Changes in the control of cell reproduction leading to cancer may be due to environmental exposure or inherited genetic flaws.

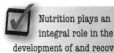
Changes in the control of cell reproduction leading to cancer may be due to environmental exposure or inherited genetic flaws.

Individuals who smoke cigarettes have an increased risk for cancer of the larynx, oral cavity, oropharynx, esophagus, lungs, bladder, pancreas, and cervix. Additional environmental carcinogens include natural and synthetic pesticides, water and air pollution, food additives, and occupational hazards.

Another source of environmental risk for cancer is ultraviolet radiation. Individuals who are chronic sunbathers or who use tanning booths are at increased risk for developing skin cancer. Other types of radiation exposure are from x-rays, radioactive materials, and atomic wastes. Oncogenic viruses also contribute to the incidence of cancer.

Genetic predisposition has been identified in several types of cancer (e.g., breast and colon). Other risk factors for cancer include race, diet, gender, age, occupation, and living environment. Sustained stress is also considered a risk factor for cancer because it affects the endocrine and immune systems. Nutrition plays an integral role in the development of and recovery from cancer.

Nutrition plays an integral role in the development of and recovery from cancer.

CONDITIONS RELATED TO THE DISEASE PROCESS OR TREATMENT

Cancer is associated with three basic nutritional outcomes: anorexia, hypermetabolic state, and negative nitrogen balance. For many individuals, weight loss and weakness are due to abnormalities in glucose and protein metabolism. Cancer patients do not produce glucose efficiently from carbohydrates and instead break down their own tissue protein and convert it to glucose. Anorexia often develops from discomfort associated with eating or digestion but may also be due to depression.

 Anorexia often develops from discomfort associated with eating or digestion but may also be due to depression.

Malabsorption develops when cancer involves the pancreas, pancreatic duct, or common bile duct; normal secretory function of digestive enzymes; and related materials such as bile salts. Individuals who experience this type of cancer are at risk for decreased prothrombin, leading to blood-clotting problems. They are also at risk for decreased digestion and absorption of fats and fat-soluble vitamins.

Vitamin D deficiency leads to decreased calcium absorption and metabolism, thus increasing the risk for osteomalacia.

Individuals who have cancer of the digestive system will likely experience malabsorption due to diarrhea, vomiting, and obstruction.

Malabsorption results in protein loss, fluid and electrolyte imbalances (especially of sodium and potassium), hormonal imbalance, and anemia. Nutritional problems also result from cancer treatment such as surgery, radiotherapy, and chemotherapy.

 Nutritional problems also result from cancer treatment such as surgery, radiotherapy, and chemotherapy.

WAYS TO ENHANCE NUTRITION

It is important to complete a personal nutrition assessment in order to provide an appropriate nutritional treatment for a cancer patient. An initial nutrition assessment is directed at developing baseline information that can be altered as necessary to meet the needs of the individual. It is important

 It is important to complete a personal nutrition assessment in order to provide an appropriate nutritional treatment for a cancer patient.

to identify the individual's needs (based on type, location, and extent of the cancer), current nutritional status, and personal desires, tolerances, and dislikes.

The amount of total dietary calories depends on the current nutritional status of the individual. If the adult has good nutritional status, about 2000 kcal is sufficient. However, if the individual is already malnourished, the calorie requirement may be as high as 3000–4000 kcal.

It is important to have adequate carbohydrate intake to prevent further tissue destruction. Ideally, carbohydrates should supply the majority of calories, and fat should account for approximately 30% or less of the intake.

Protein intake may need to be increased to meet maintenance needs, ensure adequate intake, prevent protein wasting, and provide nitrogen for healing and tissue regeneration.

Adequate vitamins and minerals are essential in nutritional therapy. Specifically, the B-complex vitamins are coenzyme agents in energy and protein metabolism. Vitamins A and C are used in tissue building. Also, vitamin A plays a role in protective cell immunity and cell differentiation. Vitamin C serves as an antioxidant, with enzymatic and immune biological functions. Vitamins A, D, and E may be useful in reducing certain oncogenes. Vitamin D also helps with calcium and phosphorus metabolism. Vitamin E protects cell wall integrity. Sufficient fluid intake is necessary. Fluids help to eliminate the breakdown products of chemotherapy agents and destroyed cancer cells. In addition, adequate fluid intake protects the urinary tract from irritation and inflammation.

Questions to Ask Cancer Patients

What is the current status of the cancer (type, location, extent)?
What are your food preferences and dislikes?
What can you tolerate in terms of amount of foods and fluids?
What are your current problems related to nutrition?
What did you eat in the past 24 hours? Is this typical?
What type of supplements have you utilized or tolerated (e.g., protein drinks, vitamins)?
What are your feelings (e.g., depression, anxiety) related to having cancer? In what ways do these feelings impact your nutritional intake?

SUGGESTIONS TO IMPROVE NUTRITIONAL INTAKE

- Develop goals related to adequate protein and calories based on individual nutrition assessment.
- Be sure that foods are presented with a variety of texture (as tolerated), color, aroma, and taste.

- Offer small, frequent foods that offer a variety and are a part of the planned nutritional goals.
- Encourage exercise before meals.
- Ensure that the environment is conducive to eating: reduce stressors, eat slowly, rest afterward.
- If individual experiences oral and throat ulcerations, provide small, frequent snacks that are bland in nature and cool in temperature.
- Provide topical anesthetic washes, sprays, or gels as needed.
- Make sure good oral hygiene is maintained.
- Check for adequate salivary secretions; offer sufficient liquid content.

CHAPTER 22 · QUESTIONS

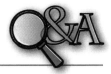

1. Which type of cancer originates from the connective tissue?
   a. Sarcoma
   b. Carcinoma
   c. Sarcoidoma
   d. Adenocarcinoma

2. Cancer is associated with which basic outcome?
   a. Anorexia
   b. Hypermetabolic state
   c. Negative nitrogen balance
   d. All of the above

3. It is important that cancer patients consume protein for what reason?
   a. To prevent protein wasting
   b. To provide nitrogen for healing
   c. To provide nitrogen for tissue replacement
   d. All of the above

4. Which vitamin plays an important role in protective cell immunity and cell differentiation?
   a. Vitamin A
   b. Vitamin B
   c. Vitamin D
   d. Vitamin E

5. Which vitamin serves as an antioxidant, enzymatic, and immune biological agent?
   a. Vitamin A
   b. Vitamin B
   c. Vitamin C
   d. Vitamin D

6. Which vitamin helps with calcium and phosphorus metabolism?
   a. Vitamin A
   b. Vitamin B
   c. Vitamin C
   d. Vitamin D

7. It is important for cancer patients to have adequate fluid intake because it offers what help?
   a. Protection against urinary tract irritation and inflammation
   b. Eliminating breakdown of products of chemotherapy
   c. None of the above
   d. A and B

8. For a patient with cancer who is already malnourished, the total daily caloric requirement may need to be how much?
   a. 1000–1500 kcal
   b. 1500–2000 kcal
   c. 2000–3000 kcal
   d. 3000–4000 kcal

9. What is the recommended percentage of fat in the diet of a patient who has cancer?
   a. 10%
   b. 15%
   c. 30%
   d. 35%

10. For the patient who has cancer, adequate carbohydrate intake is necessary for what reason?
    a. To prevent further tissue destruction
    b. To provide cell immunity
    c. To prevent cell differentiation
    d. To serve as an antioxidant

CHAPTER 22 • ANSWERS AND RATIONALES

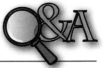

1. The answer is a.

2. The answer is d.

3. The answer is d.

4. The answer is a.

5. The answer is c.

6. The answer is d.

7. The answer is d.

8. The answer is d.

9. The answer is c.

10. The answer is a.

Statistics from the United States Department of Health and Human Services (HHS) indicate that 61% of adults in the United States were overweight or obese in 1999. Approximately 300,000 deaths each year in the United States may be attributed to obesity, and a number of diseases are associated with being overweight or obese.

Overweight and obesity are usually defined in terms of body mass index (BMI). The body mass index measures your weight in relation to your height, and is closely associated with measures of body fat. The CDC considers adults overweight if BMI is between 25 and 29.9, and obese if BMI is 30 or higher. BMI does not always accurately predict for someone with a lot of muscle or who is very short (under 5 ft) or for older people.

In 1999, it was estimated that 13% of children ages 6–11 and 14% of adolescents ages 12–19 were overweight (HHS)—an increase over the past 2 decades of almost 300%. The rates of type 2 diabetes mellitus, high cholesterol, and hypertension in children, teens, and young adults are rising significantly. The risk of an overweight or obese child or teen becoming an overweight or obese adult is 70%, which rises to 80% if one or both parents are overweight or obese.

Recommendations: Do not rely on fad or crash diets to effectively lose weight. Walk whenever possible. Be active! Reward yourself for success (without food). To prevent gradual weight gain over time, make small decreases in food and beverage calories and increase physical activity.

23

Obesity

TERMS
- [ ] body mass index (BMI)
- [ ] obesity
- [ ] health risks

Obesity is a national health problem in the United States. According to the Centers for Disease Control, since 1985 the prevalence of obesity has dramatically increased. Statistics from the United States Department of Health and Human Services (HHS) indicate that 61% of adults in the United States were overweight or obese in 1999; approximately 300,000 deaths each year in the United States may be attributed to obesity; and, diseases such as heart disease, type 2 diabetes mellitus, stroke, arthritis, certain forms of cancer, respiratory illnesses, and psychological disorders, such as depression are associated with being overweight or obese.

Genetics certainly plays a role in the development of obesity, but behavioral and environmental factors also account for much of the development and maintenance of this health risk. Metabolism, culture, behavior, and socioeconomic status must all be taken into account when trying to plan preventive actions and treatment regimens for obesity. A study estimates that U.S. medical expenditures attributed to overweight and obesity have approached $92.6 billion in 2002 (Finkelstein, Fiebelkom, and Wang, 2003).

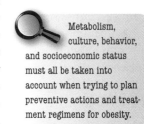

Metabolism, culture, behavior, and socioeconomic status must all be taken into account when trying to plan preventive actions and treatment regimens for obesity.

BEHAVIORS AFFECTING NUTRITION

The U.S. Surgeon General's *Call to Action to Prevent and Decrease Overweight and Obesity* (2001) simply states that overweight and obesity result from an energy imbalance. Overweight and obesity result from too many calories consumed and not enough expended. Many people in the United States are sedentary. At least 40% of adults in the United States do not participate in any leisure-time physical activity and less than one-third of adults engage in the recommended amounts, at least 30 minutes most days, of physical activity (UHHS).

Overweight and obesity result from too many calories consumed and not enough expended.

It takes 3500 kcal beyond what is needed and expended by the body to gain a pound. This can be done by drinking one 150-calorie sweetened soft drink per day above the body's needs in less than 1 month. Refer to Appendix F for a list of age-related physical activity levels and approximate calorie expenditure.

DEFINITIONS

The Centers for Disease Control and Prevention define overweight and obesity in terms of body mass index (BMI). Although BMI does not directly measure body fat, it does correlate with the amount of body fat. Other estimations of body fat include skinfold thickness, waist circumference, calculation of waist-to-hip circumference ratios, hydrostatic estimations, and imaging techniques such as ultrasound, computed tomography, and magnetic resonance imaging (MRI).

The BMI is calculated by using height and weight. (Refer to the end of the chapter for adult BMI, and to Appendix E for children and teens.) The CDC considers adults overweight if the BMI is between 25 and 29.9, and obese if the BMI is 30 or higher. Some people may have a BMI that indicates they are overweight, for instance, athletes; however, due to muscle mass they may in fact not be overweight since the BMI is a correlation with the amount of body fat.

The National Heart, Lung, and Blood Institute guidelines also recommend two other predictors of health risk associated with overweight and obesity:

- Waist circumference (abdominal fat is a predictor)
- Hypertension and physical inactivity

OBESITY AND YOUTH

Children and teens are particularly vulnerable to weight gain due to several factors, including fast foods and convenience foods with high fat and calorie content, large portion sizes (refer to Appendix G), sedentary lifestyles (watching TV, using computers, playing video games, going everywhere by car), and delivery of food to the door. In 1999, it was estimated that 13% of children 6–11 years and 14% of adolescents 12–19 years were overweight (HHS). In the last two decades, overweight and obesity of children and teens has increased, almost 300%. The risk of an overweight or obese child or teen becoming an overweight or obese adult is 70%, which rises to 80% if one or both parents are also overweight or obese.

Not only may overweight and obese children and teens become overweight and obese

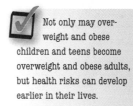
Not only may overweight and obese children and teens become overweight and obese adults, but health risks can develop earlier in their lives.

adults, but health risks can develop earlier in their lives. The rates of type 2 diabetes mellitus, high cholesterol, and hypertension in children, teens, and young adults are rising significantly. Psychological disorders such as low self-esteem and depression are also more prevalent in overweight and obese children and teens, associated with social discrimination.

The definition of overweight and obesity by the BMI takes into account body fat differences between boys and girls at various ages. (Refer to Appendix E.)

SUGGESTIONS FOR WEIGHT LOSS

- Follow the 2005 Dietary Guidelines for Americans for healthy eating and physical activity.
- Consult your health care provider and develop a goal BMI.
- Assess your health risk factors already present for comorbid diseases such as hypertension and/or diabetes, and get them under control with the assistance of a health care provider.
- Evaluate unhealthy behaviors and make contracts with yourself to change, such as stopping smoking.
- Do not rely on fad or crash diets to lose weight. For children and teens restrictive diets are not healthy because children and teens are still growing.
- Commit to healthy eating and exercise that you enjoy.
- Enlist support of family and friends.
- Walk whenever possible. Be active!
- Reward yourself for success (without food).
- Be a role model for children.
- For children and teens, enlist the aid of the health care provider and school counselor for guidance in setting goals.
- Concentrate on positive attitudes for children and teens, not on their weight.
- Show love and support for a child's or teen's progress.

KEY RECOMMENDATIONS OF THE 2005 DIETARY GUIDELINES

- To maintain body weight in a healthy range, balance calories from foods and beverages with calories expended through activity and exercise.
- To prevent gradual weight gain over time, make small decreases in food and beverage calories and increase physical activity.

RECOMMENDATIONS OF THE 2005 DIETARY GUIDELINES FOR SPECIFIC POPULATION GROUPS

- For those persons who need to lose weight, a slow and steady weight loss is the goal by decreasing caloric intake while maintaining an adequate nutrient intake and increasing physical activity.
- For children who are overweight, the goal is to reduce the rate of body weight gain while allowing growth and development. A health care provider must be consulted prior to instituting a weight-loss program for a child.
- For pregnant women, ensure appropriate weight gain as specified by a health care provider.
- For breastfeeding women, a moderate weight reduction is safe and does not compromise weight gain of the infant.
- For overweight adults and children with chronic diseases and/or those taking medication, a weight-loss program must be developed in conjunction with a health care provider to ensure appropriate management of other health conditions.

THE BODY MASS INDEX

BMI measures your weight in relation to your height and is closely associated with measures of body fat. Because BMI does not show the difference between fat and muscle, it does not always accurately predict when weight could lead to health problems. For example, someone with a lot of muscle (such as a body builder) may have a BMI in the excess weight range, but still be healthy and have little risk of developing diabetes or having a heart attack.

The BMI also may not accurately reflect body fatness in people who are very short (under 5 ft) and in older people, who tend to lose muscle mass as they age. And it may not be the best predictor of weight-related health problems among some racial and ethnic groups such as African American and Hispanic/Latino American women. But for most people, BMI is a reliable way to tell if your weight is putting your health at risk.

You can calculate your BMI using this formula:

$$\text{BMI} = \frac{\text{weight (lb)} \times 703}{\text{height squared (in.}^2)}$$

For example, for someone who is 5 ft. 7 in. tall and weighs 220 lbs, the calculation would look like this:

$$\text{BMI} = \frac{220 \text{ lb} \times 703}{67 \text{ in.} \times 67 \text{ in.}} = \frac{154{,}660}{4489} = 34.45$$

A BMI of 18.5 to 24.9 is considered healthy. A person with a BMI of 25 to 29.9 is considered overweight, and a person with a BMI of 30 or more is considered obese.

You can also find your weight group on the chart in Figure 23-1. Find your weight on the bottom of the graph. Go straight up from that point until you come to the line that matches your height. Then look to find your weight group. The higher your BMI is over 25, the greater chance you may have of developing health problems.

The chart applies to all adults. The higher weights in the healthy range apply to people with more muscle and bone, such as men. Even within the healthy range, weight gain could increase your risk for health problems.

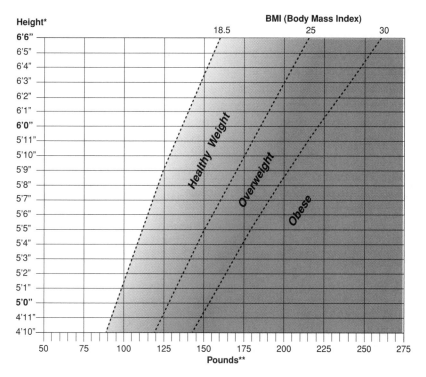

Height*   **BMI (Body Mass Index)**

* Without shoes **Without clothes

Figure 23-1 Chart for Determining BMI.

Source: Weight-control Information Network (WIN). An information service of the National Institute of Diabetes and Digestive and Kidney Diseases (NIDDK). *Weight and Waist Measurements: Tools for Adults.* http://win.niddk.nih.gov/publications/tools.htm#bodymassindex

SOURCES

Finkelstein EA, Fiebelkom IC, Wang G. National medical spending attributable to overweight and obesity: how much, and who's paying? *Health Aff.* 2003; Jan. (supple. web exclusive):W3-219–226.

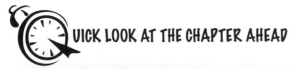

Toxic food-borne agents include bacteria, viruses, and protozoa. Symptoms are generally gastrointestinal, but fever, headache, and chills can also be present. Onset may be one hour to several days. Severe cases require hospitalization. Botulism can be fatal.

Infants, children, elderly adults, the debilitated, and those with cancer, diabetes, liver disease, hemochromatosis, stomach disease, previous surgery, a compromised immune system, or who have used steroids on a long-term basis are particularly susceptible.

For prevention, personal hygiene is a must. Hands must be washed with soap and hot water and dried thoroughly after using bathroom facilities and prior to handling food, raw or uncooked. Any person who is ill should not be handling food. Contact with the nose, mouth, or hair should be avoided. Do not taste or sample foods during preparation.

Utensils, equipment, and cutting boards should be thoroughly cleaned between uses. "Keep hot food hot and cold foods cold." Hot foods should be cooled in a cooling bath of cool water and not slow cooled on the counter.

Raw meats should not be stored for more than 7 days in the refrigerator. Raw poultry, fish, and ground meat should not be stored for more than 2 days. Ground meat may be a particular hazard. Be aware of expiration dates. Cook foods thoroughly, especially pork and pork products. Use a clean thermometer that measures the internal

24

Food Safety

TERMS
- ☐ botulism
- ☐ bacteria
- ☐ viruses
- ☐ protozoa

temperature of cooked food to make sure meat, poultry, and casseroles are cooked to the proper temperature.

When traveling, beware of contaminated water used for drinking, ice, or washing fruits and vegetables. Take your own fluids when you are not sure.

The 2005 Dietary Guidelines for Americans: Clean hands, contact surfaces, fruits, and vegetables. Separate raw, cooked, and ready-to-eat foods. Cook foods at a safe temperature. Chill or refrigerate perishable foods promptly. Infants and young children, pregnant women, older adults, and the immunocompromised should not drink or eat raw (unpasteurized) milk or any products made from unpasteurized milk, raw or partially cooked eggs, or foods containing raw eggs, raw or undercooked meat and poultry, raw or undercooked fish or shellfish, unpasteurized juices, and raw sprouts.

Food-borne illnesses not only may affect the health and lives of individuals, but the threat of bioterrorism may affect food and water supplies of thousands. Toxic food-borne agents vary, but etiologies include bacteria, viruses, and protozoa. Symptoms generally are gastrointestinal, but systemic manifestations such as fever, headache, chills can also be present in certain illnesses. Onset may be from as little as 1 hour to several days depending on the causative organism, but severe cases require hospitalization.

One of the most virulent food-borne illnesses, botulism, is often fatal.

Infants, children, elderly adults, and those who are debilitated are particularly susceptible to food-borne illness. Escherichia coliform (*E. coli*) has caused gastrointestinal illness and deaths in recent years in children in the United States and Canada. Vulnerable populations at risk to develop complications are those with diseases such as cancer, diabetes, liver disease, hemochromatosis, stomach disease, and/or previous surgery. Particularly at risk are those with compromised immune systems including those with HIV/AIDS, and those who have used steroids on a long-term basis for such diseases as arthritis or asthma.

KEY RECOMMENDATIONS OF THE 2005 DIETARY GUIDELINES

Personal hygiene is a must for prevention. Thorough handwashing is imperative prior to handling any food, raw or cooked. Hands must be washed after using bathroom facilities with soap and hot water and dried thoroughly.

> ✓ Thorough handwashing is imperative prior to handling any food, raw or cooked.

> ❗ Any person who is ill should not be handling food.

Contact with the nose, mouth, or hair for any individual, not only the sick, should be avoided if near food during storing or preparation. Tasting or sampling foods during preparation is not advised.

The food environment such as food utensils and equipment should be thoroughly cleaned between uses. Cutting boards must be adequately washed to prevent cross-contamination of foods, especially if used to prepare raw meats.

> ✓ The food environment such as food utensils and equipment should be thoroughly cleaned between uses. Cutting boards must be adequately washed to prevent cross-contamination of foods, especially if used to prepare raw meats.

The old adage, "keep hot foods hot and cold foods cold," still applies. Cooked foods should not be at a temperature of 60° to 125°F (room temperature or above) for more than 2 hours. Creamed pies, gravies, and foods containing mayonnaise are very susceptible to contamination if not refrigerated promptly. Leftovers should be reheated to 165°F to destroy vegetative bacterial cells that may have formed.

> ❗ Hot foods should be cooled in a cooling bath of cold water and not slow-cooled on the counter, since the latter provides a good medium for bacterial growth.

Raw meats should not be stored for more than 7 days in a refrigerator. Raw poultry, fish, and ground meat should not be stored for more than 2 days.

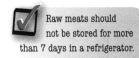

> ✓ Raw meats should not be stored for more than 7 days in a refrigerator.

Ground meat may be a particular hazard—if cutting surfaces or utensils used in processing are contaminated, the organisms may be throughout the meat and not only on the surface.

Consumers need to be aware of expiration dates on products, especially perishable items, e.g., eggs, luncheon meats, and milk products. Only food products that meet government standards for food safety should be purchased, such as USDA-inspected meats, pasteurized milk and dairy products, and fish. Foods need to be cooked thoroughly, especially pork and pork products, to prevent food-borne illnesses.

> Foods need to be cooked thoroughly, especially pork and pork products, to prevent food-borne illnesses.

If traveling, check the safety of water supplies and be prepared to bring fluids on trips, particularly outside of the United States and Canada. If the water supply is questionable, the consumer needs to be aware of situations in which contaminated water, such as melted ice, may be used for washing fruits and vegetables for salads, and avoid these foods.

The health care provider can be a resource of information as well as a teacher for prevention of food-borne illness. Opportunities for education about food safety abound in the health care setting and the community.

> The health care provider can be a resource of information as well as a teacher for prevention of food-borne illness. Opportunities for education about food safety abound in the health care setting and the community.

The 2005 Dietary Guidelines for Americans list of behaviors to prevent food safety problems include:

- cleaning hands, contact surfaces, and fruits and vegetables prior to consumption. Meat and poultry should not be washed, due to possible contamination by handling and thereby spreading bacteria to other foods.
- separating raw, cooked, and ready-to-eat foods while purchasing, preparing, or storing.
- cooking foods at a safe temperature (refer to chart).
- chilling or refrigerating perishable foods promptly.

Infants and young children, pregnant women, older adults, and those who are immunocompromised should not drink or eat raw (unpasteurized) milk or any products made from unpasteurized milk, raw or partially cooked eggs or foods containing raw eggs, raw or undercooked meat and poultry, raw or undercooked fish or shellfish, unpasteurized juices, and raw sprouts.

Pregnant women, older adults, and those who are immunocompromised should only eat deli meats and frankfurters that have been reheated to steaming hot.

TEMPERATURE RULES FOR SAFE COOKING AND HANDLING OF FOODS

Bacteria multiply rapidly between 40°F and 140°F, doubling in number in as little as 20 minutes. To keep food out of this danger zone, keep cold food cold and hot food hot.

Keep cold food in the refrigerator, in coolers, or on the service line on ice. Set your refrigerator no higher than 40°F and the freezer at 0°F.

Keep hot food in the oven, in heated chafing dishes, or in preheated steam tables, warming trays, and/or slow cookers.

Use a clean thermometer that measures the internal temperature of cooked food to make sure meat, poultry, and casseroles are cooked to the temperatures as indicated in Figure 24-1.

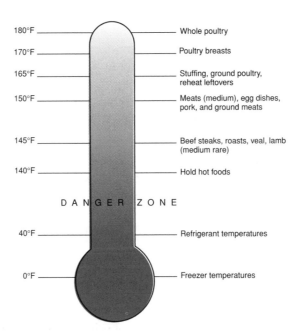

Figure 24-1 Safe cooking and holding temperatures for foods.

Source: USDA Dietary Guidelines 2005. Chapter 10, Food Safety: Figure 5 and caption. http://www.health.gov/dietaryguidelines/dga2005/document/html/chapter10.htm

Alcohol interferes with the ability of the body to digest, store, uses and excrete nutrients. Drink alcoholic beverages sensibly and in moderation (1 drink per day for women and up to 2 for men). Individuals who cannot control alcohol intake should not drink.

Those who should not drink at all: women of childbearing age who might become pregnant, pregnant and lactating women, children and adolescents, people taking medications that can interact with alcohol, who have specific medical conditions, or who participate in activities that require alertness, skill, or coordination.

Moderate alcohol consumption may reduce the risk of coronary heart disease among men older than 45 years and women older than 55 years. Individuals who consume alcohol are at increased risk for health problems. Women who drink are at a greater risk for breast cancer. A fetus exposed to alcohol during a pregnancy risks mental retardation or behavior/learning problems.

Drinking lessens nutritional intake and inhibits the digestive breakdown of food. Alcoholics are likely to get up to 50% of their total daily calories from alcohol. Alcohol can cause either hypoglycemia or hyperglycemia.

Alcohol-induced vitamin deficiencies lead to night blindness (vitamin A), softening of the bones (vitamin D), deficiencies in blood clotting (vitamin K), and wound healing and cell maintenance (vitamin B complex). Mineral deficiencies due to alcohol create decreased calcium absorption; iron

25

Alcohol

TERMS
- [ ] binge drinking
- [ ] physical dependence
- [ ] wernicke-korsafoff syndrome

deficiency; and skin lesions. Long-term alcohol use leads to vitamin A and vitamin E not being absorbed, damages the pancreas, and does neurological damage.

Standards of care and the effectiveness of nutritional therapy for the cure or treatment of alcoholism have not been established. Mega-dosing of nutrients, particularly the fat-soluble vitamins, is not advisable.

Alcohol interferes with the ability of the body to digest, store, use, and excrete nutrients. Individuals who abuse alcohol are likely to eat poorly, so their intake of vitamins and minerals is limited and often their body's ability to use the nutrients effectively is decreased.

KEY RECOMMENDATIONS

- Drink alcoholic beverages sensibly and in moderation (defined as one drink per day for women and up to two drinks per day for men).
- Individuals who cannot restrict their alcohol intake should not drink any alcohol.
- Women of childbearing age who may become pregnant, pregnant and lactating women, children and adolescents, individuals taking medications that can interact with alcohol, and those with specific medical conditions should not consume alcohol.
- Individuals who participate in activities that require alertness, skill, or coordination such as driving or operating machinery should not drink alcoholic beverages.

RISKS OF EXCESSIVE ALCOHOL CONSUMPTION

Moderate alcohol consumption may reduce the risk of coronary heart disease among men over age 45 and women over age 55, but individuals need to consider lifestyle changes such as a healthy diet, physical activity, smoking cessation, and maintenance of a healthy weight to significantly reduce the risk of cardiac disease. Individuals who consume alcohol are at increased risk for health problems. Women who drink alcohol are at a greater risk for breast cancer than women who do not drink. When a fetus is exposed to alcohol during pregnancy, there is a risk for mental retardation due to fetal alcohol syndrome or behavioral/learning problems due to fetal alcohol effect.

Moderate alcohol consumption may reduce the risk of coronary heart disease among men over age 45 and women over age 55, but individuals need to consider lifestyle changes such as a healthy diet, physical activity, smoking cessation, and maintenance of a healthy weight to significantly reduce the risk of cardiac disease.

ALCOHOL AND NUTRITION

Individuals who do not drink in moderation are likely to have their nutrition impaired at two levels. First, drinking the alcohol will lessen their nutritional intake of quality foods. Alcoholics are likely to ingest as much as 50% of their total daily calories from alcohol, with little regard for the DRI of carbohydrates, fats, proteins, vitamins, and minerals. Second, the presence of alcohol will inhibit the breakdown of food by decreasing the secretion of digestive enzymes from the pancreas, prevent the absorption of the nutrients by damaging the cells in the stomach and intestinal lining, and increase problems in transporting, storing, and excreting nutrients such as fats and vitamin A.

Even when food intake is adequate, the presence of alcohol can interfere in the regulation of glucose levels and cause either hypoglycemia or hyperglycemia. Many individuals who consume an excessive amount of calories due to alcohol may not gain excessive amounts of body weight. The effect of chronic drinking triggers a heat metabolism system rather than energy.

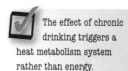

The effect of chronic drinking triggers a heat metabolism system rather than energy.

Alcohol affects protein nutrition by impairing the processing of amino acids in the small intestine and liver. Vitamins A, E, and D, along with dietary fats, are poorly absorbed. Chronic drinking also causes problems in the absorption of vitamins C, K, and B complex. Problems with vitamin deficiencies lead to conditions such as night blindness (vitamin A), softening of the bones (vitamin D), deficiencies in blood clotting (vitamin K), wound healing, and cell maintenance (vitamin B complex).

Mineral deficiencies due to alcohol create problems such as decreased calcium absorption because of fat malabsorption, iron deficiency due to gastrointestinal bleeding, and skin lesions related to zinc malabsorption.

Individuals may experience poor nutrition as a result of long-term alcohol use because vitamin A and vitamin E are not absorbed. Prolonged exposure to alcohol also damages the ability of the pancreas to function. Neurological damage (Wernicke-Korsakoff syndrome) may occur due to alcohol use.

TREATMENT OF ALCOHOLISM

No precise levels of circulating proteins, vitamins, and minerals have been established for standards of care for individuals who abuse alcohol. It is important to remember that there is little research to demonstrate effectiveness of nutritional therapy for a cure or treatment of alcoholism. In addition, it is also important to remember that mega-dosing of nutrients, particularly fat-soluble vitamins, may create an overdose.

DEFINITIONS

What's in one drink? 12 ounces of regular beer, 5 ounces of wine, 1.5 ounces of 80-proof distilled spirits.

What is moderate drinking? For women, no more than one drink a day. For men, no more than two drinks a day.

Binge drinking is generally defined as having five or more drinks on one occasion, meaning in a row or within a short period of time. Among women, binge drinking is often defined as having four or more drinks on one occasion

Heavy drinking is consuming alcohol in excess of one drink per day on average for women, and greater than two drinks per day on average for men.

Craving alcohol is a strong need, or compulsion to drink.

Loss of control is the inability to limit one's drinking on any given occasion.

Physical dependence is shown by withdrawal symptoms, such as nausea, sweating, shakiness, and anxiety, which occur when alcohol use is stopped after a period of heavy drinking.

Tolerance is the need to drink greater amounts of alcohol in order to "get high."

SOURCES

National Clearinghouse for Alcohol and Drug Information (NCADI)
http://www.niaaa.nih.gov/publications/aa22.htm
http://www/health.org/nongovpubs/aldietguide/default.aspx
http://www.cdc.gov/alcohol/factsheets/general_information.htm
http://store.health.org/catalog/facts.aspx?topic=3

In the body, water helps move nutrients throughout and remove waste products, provides heating and cooling, helps maintain appropriate acid/base balance, creates a backup system for shock absorption and temperature control for the fetus, and provides cleansing and protection.

When water intake drops, the kidneys conserve water. When there is too much water, they excrete fluid.

The usual thirst and drinking behaviors are usually sufficient to maintain normal hydration. Water, juice, milk, and other fluids without caffeine are appropriate for a healthy lifestyle. Risks for dehydration include too little water or too much of caffeinated beverages, fluids with high sugar content, and alcohol.

Key recommendations: Consume less than 2300 mg of sodium (approximately 1 tsp of salt) per day. Consume at least 4700 mg per day of potassium. Male adults over the age of 19 need to consume 3.7 L/day of water. Female adults over the age of 19 need to consume 2.7 L/day of water.

Additional risk factors for dehydration are age, obesity, heart disease, prescribed and nonprescribed drug use, alcohol use, and if already dehydrated. Keep cool during hot weather, especially if the humidity is high. In hot weather, drink 2 to 4 glasses (16–32 oz) of cool nonalcoholic fluids each hour. Avoid very cold drinks.

Signs of dehydration: thirst, nausea, headache, dizziness, weakness, difficulty breathing, difficulty speaking, mental confusion, impatience, decreased concentration, loss of appetite, stumbling, muscle spasms, and decreased urine output.

26

Fluid Balance

TERMS
- ☐ electrolytes
- ☐ dehydrates
- ☐ acid/base balance

Minerals in the body called electrolytes maintain a balance between intracellular and extracellular fluids. Water serves many functions in the body: it helps to move nutrient throughout the body and remove waste products, provides a heating and cooling capacity,

 Minerals in the body called electrolytes maintain a balance between intracellular and extracellular fluids.

and helps to maintain an appropriate acid/base balance. Water also creates a backup system for situations such as shock absorption and temperature control for the fetus, and cleansing and protection when needed.

The kidneys function to maintain fluid status in the body, e.g., when water intake is decreased, the kidneys conserve water. When there is an excess amount of water, the kidneys excrete a large volume of fluid. There is a network of osmoreceptors in the hypothalamus of the brain that are sensitive to sodium. When the sodium concentration rises, the osmoreceptors send a message to the pituitary gland to release antidiuretic hormone and this causes the kidneys to reabsorb water.

 There is a network of osmoreceptors in the hypothalamus of the brain that are sensitive to sodium. When the sodium concentration rises, the osmoreceptors send a message to the pituitary gland to release antidiuretic hormone and this causes the kidneys to reabsorb water.

The combination of thirst and drinking behaviors, especially the consumption of fluids with meals, is usually sufficient to maintain normal hydration. Purposeful drinking is warranted for individuals who are exposed to heat stress or who perform sustained vigorous activity.

Thirst is affected by taste, availability, cultural patterns, personal habits, increased osmolarity of the fluids surrounding the osmoreceptors in the hypothalamus, reduced blood volume and blood pressure, increased angiotension II, and dryness of the mouth and mucous membranes lining the esophagus.

Individuals are at risk for dehydration when they consume too little water or mostly caffeinated beverages, fluids with high sugar content, and alcohol. Individuals who take prescribed diuretic medications may experience fluid, sodium, and/or potassium imbalance, and need to be monitored carefully. To maintain a healthy lifestyle, individuals should consume mostly water, juice, milk, and other fluids without caffeine.

 To maintain a healthy lifestyle, individuals should consume mostly water, juice, milk, and other fluids without caffeine.

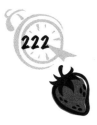

KEY RECOMMENDATIONS FOR PROPER FLUID BALANCE

- Consume less than 2300 mg of sodium (approximately 1 tsp of salt) per day.
- Consume at least 4700 mg per day of potassium.
- Male adults over the age of 19 need to consume 3.7 L/day of water.
- Female adults over the age of 19 need to consume 2.7 L/day of water.

Refer to Appendix A for a complete list of the water guidelines for all age groups.

EFFECTS OF HOT WEATHER

It is important for individuals to remember to keep cool during hot weather—especially if the humidity is high, since the body is not be able to eliminate body heat effectively. Risk factors to consider for dehydration include age, obesity, heart disease, prescribed and nonprescribed drug use, alcohol use, and if the person is already dehydrated.

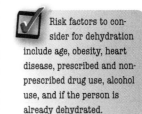
Risk factors to consider for dehydration include age, obesity, heart disease, prescribed and nonprescribed drug use, alcohol use, and if the person is already dehydrated.

It is recommended during hot weather to increase fluid intake, regardless of activity level or thirst. Individuals need to drink two to four glasses (16–32 oz) of cool nonalcoholic fluids each hour during hot weather. Avoid very cold drinks since they may cause stomach cramping. Individuals who take diuretics (water pills) need to check with their physician regarding management of fluids.

SIGNS OF DEHYDRATION

Thirst
Nausea
Headache
Dizziness

Weakness
Difficulty breathing
Difficulty speaking
Mental confusion
Impatience
Decreased concentration
Loss of appetite
Stumbling
Muscle spasms
Decreased urine output

SOURCES

Insel, P., Turner, R. E., & Ross, D. (2004). *Nutrition.* Sudbury, MA: Jones and Bartlett Publishers. Chapter 11, Water and Major Minerals.

http://www.bt.cdc.gov/disasters/extremeheat/heat_guide.asp#drink

http://www.health.gov/dietaryguidelines/dga2005

http://www.health.gov/dietaryguidelines/dga2005/edocument/html/executivesummary.htm

There are two types of eating disorders: anorexia nervosa and bulimia nervosa. A third category is any eating disorder not otherwise specified, e.g., binge eating.

An individual with anorexia nervosa refuses to maintain a normal body weight, has an intense fear of gaining weight, and has a false perception of body shape or size. Bulimia nervosa is binge eating and purging to maintain body shape and weight.

Binge eating is a lack of control over eating. The individual eats large amounts quickly even when full or not hungry, eats alone, and has feelings of disgust, guilt, and/or embarrassment.

Anorexia and bulimia can be life-threatening. Fluid and electrolyte imbalance are risks. Obesity is a risk factor for a binge eater. Vomiting affects nutrition, causes erosion of dental enamel and dental caries, and inflames the salivary glands, especially the parotid glands. Bulimia may cause gastroesophageal reflux disease (GERD), muscle weakness, fatigue, cardiac arrhythmias, and dehydration. Anorexia can bring on osteopenia and osteoporosis.

Medical and nutritional management with an interdisciplinary team are essential for the treatment of eating disorders. The individual must have a complete physical exam and health history to determine a plan of action. Lab values must be completed.

Values that may be abnormal: leukopenia, hypomagnesemia, hyponatremia, hypozincemia, hypophosphatemia, hyperamylasemia, hypochloremia, hypokalemia, elevated bicarbonate, hypercholesterolemia, hyperadrenocorticism, low T_4 and T_3, low serum estrogen levels in women, low serum testosterone levels in men.

27

Eating Disorders

TERMS
- [ ] anorexia nervosa
- [ ] bulimia nervosa
- [ ] binge eating

Eating disorders are severe disturbances in eating behavior that persist over time. There are two types of eating disorders: anorexia nervosa and bulimia nervosa. A third category in the *DSM IV-TR* is any eating disorder not otherwise specified, which includes binge eating.

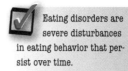

Eating disorders are severe disturbances in eating behavior that persist over time.

Anorexia nervosa is a condition in which the individual refuses to maintain a normal body weight for age and height (85%), describes an intense fear of gaining weight, and exhibits a significant disturbance in the perception of body shape or size. Another symptom is amenorrhea in postmenarcheal females with this disorder.. There are two subtypes: restricting (weight loss occurs as a result of dieting, fasting, exercise) and binge eating and purging (using vomiting, laxatives, diuretics, or enemas).

Bulimia nervosa involves binge eating and the prevention of weight gain through compensatory methods. The individual is concerned about body shape and weight. Individuals affected by bulimia will binge on different types of foods, frequently sweet, high-calorie foods. The binge will occur for a limited time, usually within a 2-hour time period. There are two subtypes: purging (regular use of laxatives, diuretics, enemas, and self-induced vomiting), and nonpurging (participates in fasting or excessive exercise, but with no regular use of laxatives, diuretics, or enemas).

Binge eating is associated with loss of control over eating and the absence of consistent use of compensatory behaviors (e.g., self-induced vomiting, laxatives, or excessive exercise). The individual demonstrates loss of control through eating quickly; eating large amounts even when full or not hungry; eating alone because of their eating habits; and feelings of disgust, guilt, and/or embarrassment related to eating.

NUTRITION AND EATING DISORDERS

There are many nutrition issues for individuals with eating disorders. It is important to remember both the cultural and age-related nutritional needs of individuals with eating disorders. Medical and nutrition management with an interdisciplinary team is essential for treatment. Nutrition issues for individuals with anorexia

It is important to remember both the cultural and age-related nutritional needs of individuals with eating disorders.

and bulimia are multiple, sometimes life-threatening:

- Fluid and electrolyte imbalance is a risk for both groups.
- Obesity is often a risk factor for the binge eater.
- Vomiting has a direct effect on nutrition.
- Gastric acid causes erosion on dental enamel and dental caries.
- Induced vomiting inflames the salivary glands, especially the parotid glands.
- Individuals with bulimia may experience gastroesophageal reflux disease (GERD), muscle weakness, fatigue, cardiac arrhythmias, and dehydration.
- Osteopenia and osteoporosis are seen in individuals with anorexia.

Even though vitamin and mineral intakes are not adequate, individuals with anorexia tend not to be deficient due to decreased metabolic need for micronutrients in a catabolic state, and in some cases the individual's taking vitamin and mineral supplements may mask the deficiencies.

MEDICAL EVALUATION OF AN EATING DISORDER

Initially, an individual with an eating disorder must have a complete physical exam and health history to determine a plan of action. Lab values must be completed. The following values may be abnormal:

- Leukopenia
- Hypomagnesemia
- Hyponatremia
- Hypozincemia
- Hypophosphatemia
- Hyperamylasemia
- Hypochloremia
- Hypokalemia
- Elevated bicarbonate
- Hypercholesterolemia
- Hyperadrenocorticism
- Hypothyroidism
- Low serum estrogen levels in women
- Low serum testosterone levels in men

SOURCES

American Psychiatric Association (4th ed.). (2000). *Diagnostic and statistical manual of mental disorders.* Washington, DC: American Psychiatric Association.

http://www.healthyplace.com/Copmmunities/Eating_Disorders/treatment_nutrition.asp

Appendix A
Dietary Reference
Intakes (DRIs)

Dietary Reference Intakes (DRIs)
Recommended Intakes for Individuals, Vitamins

Life Stage Group	Vit A (μg/d)[a]	Vit C (mg/d)	Vit D (μg/d)[b,c]	Vit E (mg/d)[d]	Vit K (μg/d)	Thiamin (mg/d)	Riboflavin (mg/d)	Niacin (mg/d)[e]	Vit B6 (mg/d)	Folate (μg/d)[f]	Vit B12 (μg/d)	Pantothenic Acid (mg/d)	Biotin (μg/d)	Choline[g] (mg/d)
Infants														
0–6 mo	400*	40*	5*	4*	2.0*	0.2*	0.3*	2*	0.1*	65*	0.4*	1.7*	5*	125*
7–12 mo	500*	50*	5*	5*	2.5*	0.3*	0.4*	4*	0.3*	80*	0.5*	1.8*	6*	150*
Children														
1–3 y	**300**	**15**	5*	**6**	30*	**0.5**	**0.5**	**6**	**0.5**	**150**	**0.9**	2*	8*	200*
4–8 y	**400**	**25**	5*	**7**	55*	**0.6**	**0.6**	**8**	**0.6**	**200**	**1.2**	3*	12*	250*
Males														
9–13 y	**600**	**45**	5*	**11**	60*	**0.9**	**0.9**	**12**	**1.0**	**300**	**1.8**	4*	20*	375*
14–18 y	**900**	**75**	5*	**15**	75*	**1.2**	**1.3**	**16**	**1.3**	**400**	**2.4**	5*	25*	550*
19–30 y	**900**	**90**	5*	**15**	120*	**1.2**	**1.3**	**16**	**1.3**	**400**	**2.4**	5*	30*	550*
31–50 y	**900**	**90**	5*	**15**	120*	**1.2**	**1.3**	**16**	**1.3**	**400**	**2.4**	5*	30*	550*
51–70 y	**900**	**90**	10*	**15**	120*	**1.2**	**1.3**	**16**	**1.7**	**400**	**2.4**[h]	5*	30*	550*
>70 y	**900**	**90**	15*	**15**	120*	**1.2**	**1.3**	**16**	**1.7**	**400**	**2.4**[h]	5*	30*	550*
Females														
9–13 y	**600**	**45**	5*	**11**	60*	**0.9**	**0.9**	**12**	**1.0**	**300**	**1.8**	4*	20*	375*
14–18 y	**700**	**65**	5*	**15**	75*	**1.0**	**1.0**	**14**	**1.2**	**400**[i]	**2.4**	5*	25*	400*
19–30 y	**700**	**75**	5*	**15**	90*	**1.1**	**1.1**	**14**	**1.3**	**400**[i]	**2.4**	5*	30*	425*
31–50 y	**700**	**75**	5*	**15**	90*	**1.1**	**1.1**	**14**	**1.3**	**400**[i]	**2.4**	5*	30*	425*
51–70 y	**700**	**75**	10*	**15**	90*	**1.1**	**1.1**	**14**	**1.5**	**400**	**2.4**[h]	5*	30*	425*
>70 y	**700**	**75**	15*	**15**	90*	**1.1**	**1.1**	**14**	**1.5**	**400**	**2.4**[h]	5*	30*	425*
Pregnancy														
14–18 y	**750**	**80**	5*	**15**	75*	**1.4**	**1.4**	**18**	**1.9**	**600**[j]	**2.6**	6*	30*	450*
19–30 y	**770**	**85**	5*	**15**	90*	**1.4**	**1.4**	**18**	**1.9**	**600**[j]	**2.6**	6*	30*	450*
31–50 y	**770**	**85**	5*	**15**	90*	**1.4**	**1.4**	**18**	**1.9**	**600**[j]	**2.6**	6*	30*	450*
Lactation														
14–18 y	**1,200**	**115**	5*	**19**	75*	**1.4**	**1.6**	**17**	**2.0**	**500**	**2.8**	7*	35*	550*
19–30 y	**1,300**	**120**	5*	**19**	90*	**1.4**	**1.6**	**17**	**2.0**	**500**	**2.8**	7*	35*	550*
31–50 y	**1,300**	**120**	5*	**19**	90*	**1.4**	**1.6**	**17**	**2.0**	**500**	**2.8**	7*	35*	550*

NOTE: This table (taken from the DRI reports, see www.nap.edu) presents Recommended Dietary Allowances (RDAs) in **bold type** and Adequate Intakes (AIs) in ordinary type followed by an asterisk (*). RDAs and AIs may both be used as goals for individual intake. RDAs are set to meet the needs of almost all (97 to 98 percent) individuals in a group. For healthy breastfed infants, the AI is the mean intake. The AI for other life stage and gender groups is believed to cover needs of all individuals in the group, but lack of data or uncertainty in the data prevent being able to specify with confidence the percentage of individuals covered by this intake.

[a] As retinol activity equivalents (RAEs). 1 RAE = 1 μg retinol, 12 μg β-carotene, 24 μg α-carotene, or 24 μg β-cryptoxanthin. The RAE for dietary provitamin A carotenoids is twofold greater than retinol equivalents (RE), whereas the RAE for preformed vitamin A is the same as RE.

[b] As cholecalciferol. 1 μg cholecalciferol = 40 IU vitamin D.

[c] In the absence of adequate exposure to sunlight.

[d] As α-tocopherol. α-Tocopherol includes RRR-α-tocopherol, the only form of α-tocopherol that occurs naturally in foods, and the 2R-stereoisomeric forms of α-tocopherol (RRR-, RSR-, RRS-, and RSS-α-tocopherol) that occur in fortified foods and supplements. It does not include the 2S-stereoisomeric forms of α-tocopherol (SRR-, SSR-, SRS-, and SSS-α-tocopherol), also found in fortified foods and supplements.

[e] As niacin equivalents (NE). 1 mg of niacin = 60 mg of tryptophan; 0–6 months = preformed niacin (not NE).

[f] As dietary folate equivalents (DFE). 1 DFE = 1 μg food folate = 0.6 μg folic acid from fortified food or as a supplement consumed with food = 0.5 μg of a supplement taken on an empty stomach.

[g] Although AIs have been set for choline, there are few data to assess whether a dietary supply of choline is needed at all stages of the life cycle, and it may be that the choline requirement can be met by endogenous synthesis at some of these stages.

[h] Because 10 to 30 percent of older people may malabsorb food-bound B12, it is advisable for those older than 50 years to meet their RDA mainly by consuming foods fortified with B12 or a supplement containing B12.

[i] In view of evidence linking folate intake with neural tube defects in the fetus, it is recommended that all women capable of becoming pregnant consume 400 μg from supplements or fortified foods in addition to intake of food folate from a varied diet.

[j] It is assumed that women will continue consuming 400 μg from supplements or fortified food until their pregnancy is confirmed and they enter prenatal care, which ordinarily occurs after the end of the periconceptional period—the critical time for formation of the neural tube.

Recommend Intakes for Individuals, Elements

Life Stage Group	Calcium (mg/d)	Chromium (µg/d)	Copper (µg/d)	Fluoride (mg/d)	Iodine (µg/d)	Iron (mg/d)	Magnesium (mg/d)	Manganese (mg/d)	Molybdenum (µg/d)	Phosphorus (mg/d)	Selenium (µg/d)	Zinc (mg/d)	Potassium (g/d)	Sodium (g/d)	Chloride (g/d)
Infants															
0–6 mo	210*	0.2*	200*	0.01*	110*	0.27*	30*	0.003*	2*	100*	15*	2*	0.4*	0.12*	0.18*
7–12 mo	270*	5.5*	220*	0.5*	130*	11	75*	0.6*	3*	275*	20*	3	0.7*	0.37*	0.57*
Children															
1–3 y	500*	11*	340	0.7*	90	7	80	1.2*	17	460	20	3	3.0*	1.0*	1.5*
4–8 y	800*	15*	440	1*	90	10	130	1.5*	22	500	30	5	3.8*	1.2*	1.9*
Males															
9–13 y	1,300*	25*	700	2*	120	8	240	1.9*	34	1,250	40	8	4.5*	1.5*	2.3*
14–18 y	1,300*	35*	890	3*	150	11	410	2.2*	43	1,250	55	11	4.7*	1.5*	2.3*
19–30 y	1,000*	35*	900	4*	150	8	400	2.3*	45	700	55	11	4.7*	1.5*	2.3*
31–50 y	1,000*	35*	900	4*	150	8	420	2.3*	45	700	55	11	4.7*	1.5*	2.3*
51–70 y	1,200*	30*	900	4*	150	8	420	2.3*	45	700	55	11	4.7*	1.3*	2.0*
> 70 y	1,200*	30*	900	4*	150	8	420	2.3*	45	700	55	11	4.7*	1.2*	1.8*
Females															
9–13 y	1,300*	21*	700	2*	120	8	240	1.6*	34	1,250	40	8	4.5*	1.5*	2.3*
14–18 y	1,300*	24*	890	3*	150	15	360	1.6*	43	1,250	55	9	4.7*	1.5*	2.3*
19–30 y	1,000*	25*	900	3*	150	18	310	1.8*	45	700	55	8	4.7*	1.5*	2.3*
31–50 y	1,000*	25*	900	3*	150	18	320	1.8*	45	700	55	8	4.7*	1.5*	2.3*
51–70 y	1,200*	20*	900	3*	150	8	320	1.8*	45	700	55	8	4.7*	1.3*	2.0*
> 70 y	1,200*	20*	900	3*	150	8	320	1.8*	45	700	55	8	4.7*	1.2*	1.8*
Pregnancy															
14–18 y	1,300*	29*	1,000	3*	220	27	400	2.0*	50	1,250	60	12	4.7*	1.5*	2.3*
19–30 y	1,000*	30*	1,000	3*	220	27	350	2.0*	50	700	60	11	4.7*	1.5*	2.3*
31–50 y	1,000*	30*	1,000	3*	220	27	360	2.0*	50	700	60	11	4.7*	1.5*	2.3*
Lactation															
14–18 y	1,300*	44*	1,300	3*	290	10	360	2.6*	50	1,250	70	13	5.1*	1.5*	2.3*
19–30 y	1,000*	45*	1,300	3*	290	9	310	2.6*	50	700	70	12	5.1*	1.5*	2.3*
31–50 y	1,000*	45*	1,300	3*	290	9	320	2.6*	50	700	70	12	5.1*	1.5*	2.3*

Note: This table presents Recommended Dietary Allowances (RDAs) in **bold type** and Adequate Intakes (AIs) in ordinary type followed by an asterisk (*). RDAs and AIs may both be used as goals for individual intake. RDAs are set to meet the needs of almost all (97 to 98 percent) individuals in a group. For healthy breastfed infants, the AI is the mean intake. The AI for other life stage and gender groups is believed to cover needs of all individuals in the group, but lack of data or uncertainty in the data prevent being able to specify with confidence the percentage of individuals covered by this intake.

Sources: *Dietary Reference Intakes for Calcium, Phosphorous, Magnesium, Vitamin D, and Fluoride* (1997); *Dietary Reference Intakes for Thiamin, Riboflavin, Niacin, Vitamin B₆, Folate, Vitamin B₁₂, Pantothenic Acid, Biotin, and Choline* (1998); *Dietary Reference Intakes for Vitamin C, Vitamin E, Selenium, and Carotenoids* (2000); *Dietary Reference Intakes for Vitamin A, Vitamin K, Arsenic, Boron, Chromium, Copper, Iodine, Iron, Manganese, Molybdenum, Nickel, Silicon, Vanadium, and Zinc* (2001); and *Dietary Reference Intakes for Water, Potassium, Sodium, Chloride, and Sulfate* (2004). These reports may be accessed via http://www.nap.edu.

Dietary Reference Intakes (DRIs): Tolerable Upper Intake Levels (UL[a]), Vitamins
Food and Nutrition Board, Institute of Medicine, National Academies

Life Stage Group	Vitamin A (µg/d)[b]	Vitamin C (mg/d)	Vitamin D (µg/d)	Vitamin E (mg/d)[c,d]	Vitamin K	Thiamin	Riboflavin	Niacin (mg/d)[d]	Vitamin B6 (mg/d)	Folate (µg/d)[d]	Vitamin B12	Pantothenic Acid	Biotin	Choline (g/d)	Carotenoids[e]
Infants															
0–6 mo	600	ND[f]	25	ND	ND	ND	ND	ND	ND	ND	ND	ND	ND	ND	ND
7–12 mo	600	ND	25	ND	ND	ND	ND	ND	ND	ND	ND	ND	ND	ND	ND
Children															
1–3 y	600	400	50	200	ND	ND	ND	10	30	300	ND	ND	ND	1.0	ND
4–8 y	900	650	50	300	ND	ND	ND	15	40	400	ND	ND	ND	1.0	ND
Males, Females															
9–13 y	1,700	1,200	50	600	ND	ND	ND	20	60	600	ND	ND	ND	2.0	ND
14–18 y	2,800	1,800	50	800	ND	ND	ND	30	80	800	ND	ND	ND	3.0	ND
19–70 y	3,000	2,000	50	1,000	ND	ND	ND	35	100	1,000	ND	ND	ND	3.5	ND
> 70 y	3,000	2,000	50	1,000	ND	ND	ND	35	100	1,000	ND	ND	ND	3.5	ND
Pregnancy															
14–18 y	2,800	1,800	50	800	ND	ND	ND	30	80	800	ND	ND	ND	3.0	ND
19–50 y	3,000	2,000	50	1,000	ND	ND	ND	35	100	1,000	ND	ND	ND	3.5	ND
Lactation															
14–18 y	2,800	1,800	50	800	ND	ND	ND	30	80	800	ND	ND	ND	3.0	ND
19–50 y	3,000	2,000	50	1,000	ND	ND	ND	35	100	1,000	ND	ND	ND	3.5	ND

[a] UL = The maximum level of daily nutrient intake that is likely to pose no risk of adverse effects. Unless otherwise specified, the UL represents total intake from food, water, and supplements. Due to lack of suitable data, ULs could not be established for vitamin K, thiamin, riboflavin, vitamin B12, pantothenic acid, biotin, carotenoids. In the absence of ULs, extra caution may be warranted in consuming levels above recommended intakes.

[b] As preformed vitamin A only.

[c] As α-tocopherol; applies to any form of supplemental α-tocopherol.

[d] The ULs for vitamin E, niacin, and folate apply to synthetic forms obtained from supplements, fortified foods, or a combination of the two.

[e] β-Carotene supplements are advised only to serve as a provitamin A source for individuals at risk of vitamin A deficiency.

[f] ND = Not determinable due to lack of data of adverse effects in this age group and concern with regard to lack of ability to handle excess amounts. Source of intake should be from food only to prevent high levels of intake.

Sources: *Dietary Reference Intakes for Calcium, Phosphorous, Magnesium, Vitamin D, and Fluoride* (1997); *Dietary Reference Intakes for Thiamin, Riboflavin, Niacin, Vitamin B6, Folate, Vitamin B12, Pantothenic Acid, Biotin, and Choline* (1998); *Dietary Reference Intakes for Vitamin C, Vitamin E, Selenium, and Carotenoids* (2000); and *Dietary Reference Intakes for Vitamin A, Vitamin K, Arsenic, Boron, Chromium, Copper, Iodine, Iron, Manganese, Molybdenum, Nickel, Silicon, Vanadium, and Zinc* (2001). These reports may be accessed via http://www.nap.edu.

Dietary Reference Intakes (DRIs): Tolerable Upper Intake Levels (UL[a]), Elements
Food and Nutrition Board, Institute of Medicine, National Academies

Life Stage Group	Arsenic[b]	Boron (mg/d)	Calcium (g/d)	Chromium	Copper (μg/d)	Fluoride (mg/d)	Iodine (μg/d)	Iron (mg/d)	Magnesium (mg/d)[c]	Manganese (mg/d)	Molybdenum (μg/d)	Nickel (mg/d)	Phosphorus (g/d)	Potassium	Selenium (μg/d)	Silicon[d]	Sulfate	Vanadium (mg/d)[e]	Zinc (mg/d)	Sodium (g/d)	Chloride (g/d)
Infants																					
0–6 mo	ND[f]	ND	ND	ND	ND	0.7	ND	40	ND	ND	ND	ND	ND	ND	45	ND	ND	ND	4	ND	ND
7–12 mo	ND	ND	ND	ND	ND	0.9	ND	40	ND	ND	ND	ND	ND	ND	60	ND	ND	ND	5	ND	ND
Children																					
1–3 y	ND	3	2.5	ND	1,000	1.3	200	40	65	2	300	0.2	3	ND	90	ND	ND	ND	7	1.5	2.3
4–8 y	ND	6	2.5	ND	3,000	2.2	300	40	110	3	600	0.3	3	ND	150	ND	ND	ND	12	1.9	2.9
Males, Females																					
9–13 y	ND	11	2.5	ND	5,000	10	600	40	350	6	1,100	0.6	4	ND	280	ND	ND	ND	23	2.2	3.4
14–18 y	ND	17	2.5	ND	8,000	10	900	45	350	9	1,700	1.0	4	ND	400	ND	ND	ND	34	2.3	3.6
19–70 y	ND	20	2.5	ND	10,000	10	1,100	45	350	11	2,000	1.0	4	ND	400	ND	ND	1.8	40	2.3	3.6
>70 y	ND	20	2.5	ND	10,000	10	1,100	45	350	11	2,000	1.0	3	ND	400	ND	ND	1.8	40	2.3	3.6
Pregnancy[e]																					
14–18 y	ND	17	2.5	ND	8,000	10	900	45	350	9	1,700	1.0	3.5	ND	400	ND	ND	ND	34	2.3	3.6
19–50 y	ND	20	2.5	ND	10,000	10	1,100	45	350	11	2,000	1.0	3.5	ND	400	ND	ND	ND	40	2.3	3.6
Lactation																					
14–18 y	ND	17	2.5	ND	8,000	10	900	45	350	9	1,700	1.0	4	ND	400	ND	ND	ND	34	2.3	3.6
19–50 y	ND	20	2.5	ND	10,000	10	1,100	45	350	11	2,000	1.0	4	ND	400	ND	ND	ND	40	2.3	3.6

[a] UL = The maximum level of daily nutrient intake that is likely to pose no risk of adverse effects. Unless otherwise specified, the UL represents total intake from food, water, and supplements. Due to lack of suitable data, ULs could not be established for arsenic, chromium, silicon, potassium, and sulfate. In the absence of ULs, extra caution may be warranted in consuming levels above recommended intakes.

[b] Although the UL was not determined for arsenic, there is no justification for adding arsenic to food or supplements.

[c] The ULs for magnesium represent intake from a pharmacological agent only and do not include intake from food and water.

[d] Although silicon has not been shown to cause adverse effects in humans, there is no justification for adding silicon to supplements.

[e] Although vanadium in food has not been shown to cause adverse effects in humans, there is no justification for adding vanadium to food and vanadium supplements should be used with caution. The UL is based on adverse effects in laboratory animals and this data could be used to set a UL for adults but not children and adolescents.

[f] ND = Not determinable due to lack of data of adverse effects in this age group and concern with regard to lack of ability to handle excess amounts. Source of intake should be from food only to prevent high levels of intake.

Sources: *Dietary Reference Intakes for Calcium, Phosphorous, Magnesium, Vitamin D, and Fluoride* (1997); *Dietary Reference Intakes for Thiamin, Riboflavin, Niacin, Vitamin B6, Folate, Vitamin B12, Pantothenic Acid, Biotin, and Choline* (1998); *Dietary Reference Intakes for Vitamin C, Vitamin E, Selenium, and Carotenoids* (2000); *Dietary Reference Intakes for Vitamin A, Vitamin K, Arsenic, Boron, Chromium, Copper, Iodine, Iron, Manganese, Molybdenum, Nickel, Silicon, Vanadium, and Zinc* (2001); and *Dietary Reference Intakes for Water, Potassium, Sodium, Chloride, and Sulfate* (2004). These reports may be accessed via http://www.nap.edu.

Dietary Reference Intakes (DRIs): Estimated Energy Requirements (EER) for Men and Women
30 Years of Age[a]
Food and Nutrition Board, Institute of Medicine, National Academies

Height (m [in])	PAL[b]	Weight for BMI[c] of 18.5 kg/m² (kg [lb])	Weight for BMI of 24.99 kg/m² (kg [lb])	EER, Men[d] (kcal/day)		EER, Women[d] (kcal/day)	
				BMI of 18.5 kg/m²	BMI of 24.99 kg/m²	BMI of 18.5 kg/m²	BMI of 24.99 kg/m²
1.50 (59)	Sedentary	41.6 (92)	56.2 (124)	1,848	2,080	1,625	1,762
	Low active			2,009	2,267	1,803	1,956
	Active			2,215	2,506	2,025	2,198
	Very active			2,554	2,898	2,291	2,489
1.65 (65)	Sedentary	50.4 (111)	68.0 (150)	2,068	2,349	1,816	1,982
	Low active			2,254	2,566	2,016	2,202
	Active			2,490	2,842	2,267	2,477
	Very active			2,880	3,296	2,567	2,807
1.80 (71)	Sedentary	59.9 (132)	81.0 (178)	2,301	2,635	2,015	2,211
	Low active			2,513	2,884	2,239	2,459
	Active			2,782	3,200	2,519	2,769
	Very active			3,225	3,720	2,855	3,141

[a] For each year below 30, add 7 kcal/day for women and 10 kcal /day for men. For each year above 30, subtract 7 kcal/day for women and 10 kcal/day for men.
[b] PAL = physical activity level.
[c] BMI = body mass index.
[d] Derived from the following regression equations based on doubly labeled water data:

Adult man: $EER = 662 - 9.53 \times age\ (y) + PA \times (15.91 \times wt\ [kg] + 539.6 \times ht\ [m])$
Adult woman: $EER = 354 - 6.91 \times age\ (y) + PA \times (9.36 \times wt\ [kg] + 726 \times ht\ [m])$

Where PA refers to coefficient for PAL

PAL = total energy expenditure ÷ basal energy expenditure

PA = 1.0 if PAL ≥ 1.0 < 1.4 (sedentary)
PA = 1.12 if PAL ≥ 1.4 < 1.6 (low active)
PA = 1.27 if PAL ≥ 1.6 < 1.9 (active)
PA = 1.45 if PAL ≥ 1.9 < 2.5 (very active)

Dietary Reference Intakes (DRIs): Acceptable Macronutrient Distribution Ranges
Food and Nutrition Board, Institute of Medicine, National Academies

Macronutrient	Range (percent of energy)		
	Children, 1–3 y	Children, 4–18 y	Adults
Fat	30–40	25–35	20–35
n-6 polyunsaturated fatty acids[a] (linoleic acid)	5–10	5–10	5–10
n-3 polyunsaturated fatty acids[a] (α-linolenic acid)	0.6–1.2	0.6–1.2	0.6–1.2
Carbohydrate	45–65	45–65	45–65
Protein	5–20	10–30	10–35

[a] Approximately 10% of the total can come from longer-chain n-3 or n-6 fatty acids.

Source: *Dietary Reference Intakes for Energy, Carbohydrate, Fiber, Fat, Fatty Acids, Cholesterol, Protein, and Amino Acids* (2002).

Recommended Intakes for Individuals, Macronutrients

Life Stage Group	Total Water[a] (L/d)	Carbohydrate (g/d)	Total Fiber (g/d)	Fat (g/d)	Linoleic Acid (g/d)	α-Linolenic Acid (g/d)	Protein[b] (g/d)
Infants							
0–6 mo	0.7*	60*	ND	31*	4.4*	0.5*	9.1*
7–12 mo	0.8*	95*	ND	30*	4.6*	0.5*	**11.0**[c]
Children							
1–3 y	1.3*	**130**	19*	ND	7*	0.7*	**13**
4–8 y	1.7*	**130**	25*	ND	10*	0.9*	**19**
Males							
9–13 y	2.4*	**130**	31*	ND	12*	1.2*	**34**
14–18 y	3.3*	**130**	38*	ND	16*	1.6*	**52**
19–30 y	3.7*	**130**	38*	ND	17*	1.6*	**56**
31–50 y	3.7*	**130**	38*	ND	17*	1.6*	**56**
51–70 y	3.7*	**130**	30*	ND	14*	1.6*	**56**
> 70 y	3.7*	**130**	30*	ND	14*	1.6*	**56**
Females							
9–13 y	2.1*	**130**	26*	ND	10*	1.0*	**34**
14–18 y	2.3*	**130**	26*	ND	11*	1.1*	**46**
19–30 y	2.7*	**130**	25*	ND	12*	1.1*	**46**
31–50 y	2.7*	**130**	25*	ND	12*	1.1*	**46**
51–70 y	2.7*	**130**	21*	ND	11*	1.1*	**46**
> 70 y	2.7*	**130**	21*	ND	11*	1.1*	**46**
Pregnancy							
14–18 y	3.0*	**175**	28*	ND	13*	1.4*	**71**
19–30 y	3.0*	**175**	28*	ND	13*	1.4*	**71**
31–50 y	3.0*	**175**	28*	ND	13*	1.4*	**71**
Lactation							
14–18 y	3.8*	**210**	29*	ND	13*	1.3*	**71**
19–30 y	3.8*	**210**	29*	ND	13*	1.3*	**71**
31–50 y	3.8*	**210**	29*	ND	13*	1.3*	**71**

Note: This table presents Recommended Dietary Allowances (RDAs) in **bold** type and Adequate Intakes (AIs) in ordinary type followed by an asterisk (*). RDAs and AIs may both be used as goals for individual intake. RDAs are set to meet the needs of almost all (97 to 98 percent) individuals in a group. For healthy infants fed human milk, the AI is the mean intake. The AI for other life stage and gender groups is believed to cover the needs of all individuals in the group, but lack of data or uncertainty in the data prevent being able to specify with confidence the percentage of individuals covered by this intake.
[a] *Total* water includes all water contained in food, beverages, and drinking water.
[b] Based on 0.8 g/kg body weight for the reference body weight.
[c] Change from 13.5 in prepublication copy due to calculation error.
Food and Nutrition Board, Institute of Medicine, National Academies.

Additional Macronutrient Recommendations

Macronutrient	Recommendation
Dietary cholesterol	As low as possible while consuming a nutritionally adequate diet
Trans fatty acids	As low as possible while consuming a nutritionally adequate diet
Saturated fatty acids	As low as possible while consuming a nutritionally adequate diet
Added sugars	Limit to no more than 25% of total energy

Source: *Dietary Reference Intakes for Energy, Carbohydrate, Fiber, Fat, Fatty Acids, Cholesterol, Protein, and Amino Acids* (2002). Food and Nutrition Board, Institute of Medicine, National Academies.

Dietary Reference Intakes (DRIs): Estimated Average Requirements for Groups
Food and Nutrition Board, Institute of Medicine, National Academies

Life Stage Group	CHO (g/d)	Protein (g/d)a	Vit A (μg/d)b	Vit C (mg/d)	Vit E (mg/d)d	Thiamin (mg/d)	Riboflavin (mg/d)	Niacin (mg/d)d	Vit B6 (mg/d)	Folate (μg/d)b	Vit B12 (μg/d)	Copper (μg/d)	Iodine (μg/d)	Iron (mg/d)	Magnesium (mg/d)	Molybdenum (μg/d)	Phosphorus (mg/d)	Selenium (μg/d)	Zinc (mg/d)
Infants																			
7–12 mo		9*												6.9					2.5
Children																			
1–3 y	100	11	210	13	5	0.4	0.4	5	0.4	120	0.7	260	65	3.0	65	13	380	17	2.5
4–8 y	100	15	275	22	6	0.5	0.5	6	0.5	160	1.0	340	65	4.1	110	17	405	23	4.0
Males																			
9–13 y	100	27	445	39	9	0.7	0.8	9	0.8	250	1.5	540	73	5.9	200	26	1,055	35	7.0
14–18 y	100	44	630	63	12	1.0	1.1	12	1.1	330	2.0	685	95	7.7	340	33	1,055	45	8.5
19–30 y	100	46	625	75	12	1.0	1.1	12	1.1	320	2.0	700	95	6	330	34	580	45	9.4
31–50 y	100	46	625	75	12	1.0	1.1	12	1.1	320	2.0	700	95	6	350	34	580	45	9.4
51–70 y	100	46	625	75	12	1.0	1.1	12	1.4	320	2.0	700	95	6	350	34	580	45	9.4
>70 y	100	46	625	75	12	1.0	1.1	12	1.4	320	2.0	700	95	6	350	34	580	45	9.4
Females																			
9–13 y	100	28	420	39	9	0.7	0.8	9	0.8	250	1.5	540	73	5.7	200	26	1,055	35	7.0
14–18 y	100	38	485	56	12	0.9	0.9	11	1.0	330	2.0	685	95	7.9	300	33	1,055	45	7.3
19–30 y	100	38	500	60	12	0.9	0.9	11	1.1	320	2.0	700	95	8.1	255	34	580	45	6.8
31–50 y	100	38	500	60	12	0.9	0.9	11	1.1	320	2.0	700	95	8.1	265	34	580	45	6.8
51–70 y	100	38	500	60	12	0.9	0.9	11	1.3	320	2.0	700	95	5	265	34	580	45	6.8
>70 y	100	38	500	60	12	0.9	0.9	11	1.3	320	2.0	700	95	5	265	34	580	45	6.8
Pregnancy																			
14–18 y	135	50	530	66	12	1.2	1.2	14	1.6	520	2.2	785	160	23	335	40	1,055	49	10.5
19–30 y	135	50	550	70	12	1.2	1.2	14	1.6	520	2.2	800	160	22	290	40	580	49	9.5
31–50 y	135	50	550	70	12	1.2	1.2	14	1.6	520	2.2	800	160	22	300	40	580	49	9.5
Lactation																			
14–18 y	160	60	885	96	16	1.2	1.3	13	1.7	450	2.4	985	209	7	300	35	1,055	59	10.9
19–30 y	160	60	900	100	16	1.2	1.3	13	1.7	450	2.4	1,000	209	6.5	255	36	580	59	10.4
31–50 y	160	60	900	100	16	1.2	1.3	13	1.7	450	2.4	1,000	209	6.5	265	36	580	59	10.4

Note: This table presents Estimated Average Requirements (EARs), which serve two purposes: for assessing adequacy of population intakes, and as the basis for calculating Recommended Dietary Allowances (RDAs) for individuals for those nutrients. EARs have not been established for vitamin D, vitamin K, pantothenic acid, biotin, choline, calcium, chromium, fluoride, manganese, or other nutrients not yet evaluated via the DRI process.

a For individual at reference weight. *indicates change from prepublication copy due to calculation error.

b As retinol activity equivalents (RAEs). 1 RAE = 1 μg retinol, 12 μg β-carotene, 24 μg α-carotene, or 24 μg β-cryptoxanthin. The RAE for dietary provitamin A carotenoids is two-fold greater than retinol equivalents (RE), whereas the RAE for preformed vitamin A is the same as RE.

c As α-tocopherol. α-Tocopherol includes RRR-α-tocopherol, the only form of α-tocopherol that occurs naturally in foods, and the 2R-stereoisomeric forms of α-tocopherol (RRR-, RSR-, RRS-, and RSS-α-tocopherol) that occur in fortified foods and supplements. It does not include the 2S-stereoisomeric forms of α-tocopherol (SRR-, SSR-, SRS-, and SSS-α-tocopherol), also found in fortified foods and supplements.

d As niacin equivalents (NE). 1 mg of niacin = 60 mg of tryptophan.

e As dietary folate equivalents (DFE). 1 DFE = 1 μg food folate = 0.6 μg of folic acid from fortified food or as a supplement consumed with food = 0.5 μg of a supplement taken on an empty stomach.

Sources: *Dietary Reference Intakes for Calcium, Phosphorous, Magnesium, Vitamin D, and Fluoride* (1997); *Dietary Reference Intakes for Thiamin, Riboflavin, Niacin, Vitamin B6, Folate, Vitamin B12, Pantothenic Acid, Biotin, and Choline* (1998); *Dietary Reference Intakes for Vitamin C, Vitamin E, Selenium, and Carotenoids* (2000); *Dietary Reference Intakes for Vitamin A, Vitamin K, Arsenic, Boron, Chromium, Copper, Iodine, Iron, Manganese, Molybdenum, Nickel, Silicon, Vanadium, and Zinc* (2001), and *Dietary Reference Intakes for Energy, Carbohydrate, Fiber, Fat, Fatty Acids, Cholesterol, Protein, and Amino Acids* (2002). These reports may be accessed via http://www.nap.edu.

Appendix B
Sample Menus for a 2000-Calorie Food Pattern

Sample Menus for a 2000-Calorie Food Pattern

Averaged over a week, this seven-day menu provides all of the recommended amounts of nutrients and food from each food group.

Food Group		Daily Average Over One Week
GRAINS	Total Grains (oz eq)	6.0
	Whole Grains	3.4
	Refined Grains	2.6
VEGETABLES*	Total Veg* (cups)	2.6
FRUITS	Fruits (cups)	2.1
MILK	Milk (cups)	3.1
MEAT & BEANS	Meat/Beans (oz eq)	5.6
OILS	Oils (tsp/grams) 7.2 tsp/32.4 g	

*Vegetable subgroups (weekly totals)

Dk-Green Veg (cups)	3.3
Orange Veg (cups)	2.3
Beans/Peas (cups)	3.0
Starchy Veg (cups)	3.4
Other Veg (cups)	6.6

Nutrient	Daily Average Over One Week
Calories	1994
Protein, g	98
Protein, % kcal	20
Carbohydrate, g	264
Carbohydrate, % kcal	53
Total fat, g	67
Total fat, % kcal	30
Saturated fat, g	16
Saturated fat, % kcal	7.0
Monounsaturated fat, g	23
Polyunsaturated fat, g	23
Linoleic Acid, g	21
Alpha-linolenic Acid, g	1.1
Cholesterol, mg	207
Total dietary fiber, g	31
Potassium, mg	4715
Sodium, mg*	1948
Calcium, mg	1389
Magnesium, mg	432
Copper, mg	1.9
Iron, mg	21
Phosphorus, mg	1830
Zinc, mg	14
Thiamin, mg	1.9
Riboflavin, mg	2.5
Niacin Equivalents, mg	24
Vitamin B_6, mg	2.9
Vitamin B_{12}, mcg	18.4
Vitamin C, mg	190
Vitamin E, mg (AT)	18.9
Vitamin A, mcg (RAE)	1430
Dietary Folate Equivalents, mcg	558

* Starred items are foods that are labeled as no-salt-added, low-sodium, or low-salt versions of the foods. They can also be prepared from scratch with little or no added salt. All other foods are regular commercial products that contain variable levels of sodium. Average sodium level of the 7-day menu assumes no salt added in cooking or at the table.

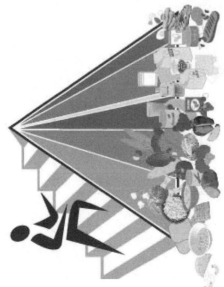

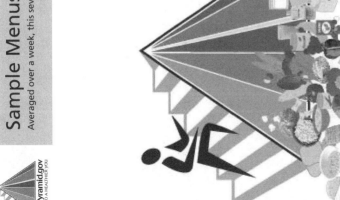

MyPyramid.gov
STEPS TO A HEALTHIER YOU

Sample Menus for a 2000-Calorie Food Pattern

Averaged over a week, this seven-day menu provides all of the recommended amounts of nutrients and food from each food group.
(Italicized foods are part of the dish or food that precedes it.)

MyPyramid.gov
STEPS TO A HEALTHIER YOU

Day 1

BREAKFAST

Breakfast burrito
1 flour tortilla (7" diameter)
1 scrambled egg (in 1 tsp soft margarine)
*1/3 cup black beans**
2 tbsp salsa
1 cup orange juice
1 cup fat-free milk

LUNCH

Roast beef sandwich
1 whole grain sandwich bun
3 ounces lean roast beef
2 slices tomato
1/4 cup shredded romaine lettuce
1/8 cup sautéed mushrooms (in 1 tsp oil)
1 1/2 ounce part-skim mozzarella cheese
1 tsp yellow mustard
3/4 cup baked potato wedges*
1 tbsp ketchup
1 unsweetened beverage

DINNER

Stuffed broiled salmon
5 ounces salmon filet
1 ounce bread stuffing mix
1 tbsp chopped onions
1 tbsp diced celery
2 tsp canola oil
1/2 cup saffron (white) rice
1 ounce slivered almonds
1/2 cup steamed broccoli
1 tsp soft margarine
1 cup fat-free milk

SNACKS

1 cup cantaloupe

Day 2

BREAKFAST

Hot cereal
1/2 cup cooked oatmeal
2 tbsp raisins
1 tsp soft margarine
1/2 cup fat-free milk
1 cup orange juice

LUNCH

Taco salad
2 ounces tortilla chips
2 ounces ground turkey, sautéed in 2 tsp sunflower oil
*1/2 cup black beans**
1/2 cup iceberg lettuce
2 slices tomato
1 ounce low-fat cheddar cheese
2 tbsp salsa
1/2 cup avocado
1 tsp lime juice
1 unsweetened beverage

DINNER

Spinach lasagna
1 cup lasagna noodles, cooked (2 oz dry)
2/3 cup cooked spinach
1/2 cup ricotta cheese
*1/2 cup tomato sauce tomato bits**
1 ounce part-skim mozzarella cheese
1 ounce whole wheat dinner roll
1 cup fat-free milk

SNACKS

1/2 ounce dry-roasted almonds*
1/4 cup pineapple
2 tbsp raisins

Day 3

BREAKFAST

Cold cereal
1 cup bran flakes
1 cup fat-free milk
1 small banana
1 slice whole wheat toast
1 tsp soft margarine
1 cup prune juice

LUNCH

Tuna fish sandwich
2 slices rye bread
3 ounces tuna (packed in water, drained)
2 tsp mayonnaise
1 tbsp diced celery
1/4 cup shredded romaine lettuce
2 slices tomato
1 medium pear
1 cup fat-free milk

DINNER

Roasted chicken breast
*3 ounces boneless skinless chicken breast**
1 large baked sweet potato
1/2 cup peas and onions
1 tsp soft margarine
1 ounce whole wheat dinner roll
1 tsp soft margarine
1 cup leafy greens salad
3 tsp sunflower oil and vinegar dressing

SNACKS

1/4 cup dried apricots
1 cup low-fat fruited yogurt

Day 4

BREAKFAST

1 whole wheat English muffin
2 tsp soft margarine
1 tbsp jam or preserves
1 medium grapefruit
1 hard-cooked egg
1 unsweetened beverage

LUNCH

White bean-vegetable soup
1 1/4 cup chunky vegetable soup
*1/2 cup white beans**
2 ounce breadstick
8 baby carrots
1 cup fat-free milk

DINNER

Rigatoni with meat sauce
1 cup rigatoni pasta (2 ounces dry)
*1/2 cup tomato sauce tomato bits**
2 ounces extra lean cooked ground beef (sautéed in 2 tsp vegetable oil)
3 tbsp grated Parmesan cheese
Spinach salad
1 cup baby spinach leaves
1/2 cup tangerine slices
1/2 ounce chopped walnuts
3 tsp sunflower oil and vinegar dressing
1 cup fat-free milk

SNACKS

1 cup low-fat fruited yogurt

Sample Menus for a 2000-Calorie Food Pattern

Averaged over a week, this seven-day menu provides all of the recommended amounts of nutrients and food from each food group.
(Italicized foods are part of the dish or food that preceeds it.)

MyPyramid.gov
STEPS TO A HEALTHIER YOU

* Starred items are foods that are labeled as no-salt-added, low-sodium, or low-salt versions of the foods. They can also be prepared from scratch with little or no added salt. All other foods are regular commercial products that contain variable levels of sodium. Average sodium level of the 7-day menu assumes no salt added in cooking or at the table

Day 5

BREAKFAST

Cold cereal
1 cup puffed wheat cereal
1 tbsp raisins
1 cup fat-free milk
1 small banana
1 slice whole wheat toast
1 tsp soft margarine
1 tsp jelly

LUNCH

Smoked turkey sandwich
2 ounces whole wheat pita bread
1/4 cup romaine lettuce
2 slices tomato
3 ounces sliced smoked turkey breast*
1 tbsp mayo-type salad dressing
1 tsp yellow mustard
1/2 cup apple slices
1 cup tomato juice*

DINNER

Grilled top loin steak
5 ounces grilled top loin steak
3/4 cup mashed potatoes
2 tsp soft margarine
1/2 cup steamed carrots
2 ounces whole wheat dinner roll
1 tsp soft margarine
1 cup fat-free milk

SNACKS

1 cup low-fat fruited yogurt

Day 6

BREAKFAST

French toast
2 slices whole wheat French toast
2 tsp soft margarine
2 tbsp maple syrup
1/2 medium grapefruit
1 cup fat-free milk

LUNCH

Vegetarian chili on baked potato
1 cup kidney beans*
1/2 cup tomato sauce w/ tomato tidbits*
3 tbsp chopped onions
1 ounce lowfat cheddar cheese
1 tsp vegetable oil
1 medium baked potato
1/2 cup cantaloupe
3/4 cup lemonade

DINNER

Hawaiian pizza
2 slices cheese pizza
1 ounce Canadian bacon
1/4 cup pineapple
2 tbsp mushrooms
2 tbsp chopped onions
Green salad
1 cup leafy greens
3 tsp sunflower oil and vinegar dressing
1 cup fat-free milk

SNACKS

5 whole wheat crackers*
1/8 cup hummus
1/2 cup fruit cocktail (in water or juice)

Day 7

BREAKFAST

Pancakes
3 buckwheat pancakes
2 tsp soft margarine
3 tbsp maple syrup
1/2 cup strawberries
3/4 cup honeydew melon
1/2 cup fat-free milk

LUNCH

Manhattan clam chowder
3 ounces canned clams (drained)
3/4 cup mixed vegetables
1 cup canned tomatoes*
10 whole wheat crackers*
1 medium orange
1 cup fat-free milk

DINNER

Vegetable stir-fry
4 ounces tofu (firm)
1/4 cup green and red bell peppers
1/2 cup bok choy
2 tbsp vegetable oil
1 cup brown rice
1 cup lemon-flavored iced tea

SNACKS

1 ounce sunflower seeds*
1 large banana
1 cup low-fat fruited yogurt

Appendix C
Eating Patterns

Table C-1 The DASH Eating Plan at 1600-, 2000-, 2600-, and 3100-Calorie Levels[a]

The number of daily servings in a food group vary, depending on caloric needs (see Table C-2). This chart can aid in planning menus and food selection in restaurants and grocery stores.

Food Groups	1600 Calories	2000 Calories	2600 Calories	3100 Calories	Serving Sizes	Examples and Notes	Significance of Each Food Group to the DASH Eating Plan
Grains[b]	6 servings	7–8 servings	10–11 servings	12–13 servings	1 slice bread 1 oz dry cereal ½ cup cooked rice, pasta, or cereal[c]	Whole-wheat bread, English muffin, pita, bread, bagel, cereals, grits, oatmeal, crackers, unsalted pretzels, and popcorn	Major sources of energy and fiber
Vegetables	3–4 servings	4–5 servings	5–6 servings	6 servings	1 cup raw leafy vegetable ½ cup cooked vegetable 6 oz vegetable juice	Tomatoes, potatoes, carrots, green peas, squash, broccoli, turnip greens, collards, kale, spinach, artichokes, green beans, lima beans, sweet potatoes	Rich sources of potassium, magnesium, and fiber

Food Groups	1600 Calories	2000 Calories	2600 Calories	3100 Calories	Serving Sizes	Examples and Notes	Significance of Each Food Group to the DASH Eating Plan
Fruits	4 servings	4–5 servings	5–6 servings	6 servings	6 oz fruit juice 1 medium fruit ¼ cup dried fruit ½ cup fresh, frozen, or canned fruit	Apricots, bananas, dates, grapes, oranges, orange juice, grapefruit, grapefruit juice, mangoes, melons, peaches, pineapples, prunes, raisins, strawberries, tangerines	Important sources of potassium, magnesium, and fiber
Low-fat or fat-free dairy foods	2–3 servings	2–3 servings	3 servings	3–4 servings	8 oz milk 1 cup yogurt 1½ oz cheese	Fat-free or low-fat milk, fat-free or low-fat buttermilk, fat-free or low-fat regular or frozen yogurt, low-fat and fat-free cheese	Major sources of calcium and protein
Meat, poultry, fish	1–2 servings	2 or less servings	2 servings	2–3 servings	3 oz cooked meats, poultry, or fish	Select only lean; trim away visible fats; broil, roast, or boil instead of frying; remove skin from poultry	Rich sources of protein and magnesium
Nuts, seeds, legumes	3–4 servings/week	4–5 servings/week	1 serving	1 serving	⅓ cup or 1½ oz nuts 2 tbsp or ½ oz seeds ½ cup cooked dry beans or peas	Almonds, filberts, mixed nuts, peanuts, walnuts, sunflower seeds, kidney beans, lentils	Rich sources of energy, magnesium, potassium, protein, and fiber

Food Groups	1600 Calories	2000 Calories	2600 Calories	3100 Calories	Serving Sizes	Examples and Notes	Significance of Each Food Group to the DASH Eating Plan
Fat and oils[d]	2 servings	2–3 servings	3 servings	4 servings	1 tsp soft margarine 1 tbsp low-fat mayonnaise 2 tbsp light salad dressing 1 tsp vegetable oil	Soft margarine, low-fat mayonnaise, light salad dressing, vegetable oil (such as olive, corn, canola, or safflower)	DASH has 27% of calories as fat (low in saturated fat), including fat in or added to foods
Sweets	0 servings	5 servings/ week	2 servings	2 servings	1 tbsp sugar 1 tbsp jelly or jam ½ oz jelly beans 8 oz lemonade	Maple syrup, sugar, jelly, jam, fruit-flavored gelatin, jelly beans, hard candy, fruit punch sorbet, ices	Sweets should be low in fat

[a] Karanja, N.M., et al. NIH publication No. 03-4082. *JADA* 8:S19–27, 1999.

[b] Whole grains are recommended for most servings to meet fiber recommendations.

[c] Equals ½–1¼ cups, depending on cereal type. Check the product's nutrition facts label.

[d] Fat content changes serving counts for fats and oils: For example, 1 tbsp of regular salad dressing equals 1 serving; 1 tbsp of a low-fat dressing equals ½ serving; 1 tbsp of a fat-free dressing equals 0 servings.

From: *USDA Dietary Guidelines for Americans 2005.* Appendix A: Eating Patterns. http://www.health.gov/dietaryguidelines/dga2005/document/html/appendixA.htm

Table C-2 USDA Food Guide

The suggested amounts of food to consume from the basic food groups, subgroups, and oils to meet recommended nutrient intakes at 12 different calorie levels. Nutrient and energy contributions from each group are calculated according to the nutrient-dense forms of foods in each group (e.g., lean meats and fat-free milk). The table also shows the discretionary calorie allowance that can be accommodated within each calorie level, in addition to the suggested amounts of nutrient-dense forms of foods in each group.

Daily Amount of Food from Each Group (vegetable subgroup amounts are per week)

Calorie Level	1000	1200	1400	1600	1800	2000
Food Group[1]	Food group amounts shown in cup (c) or ounce-equivalents (oz-eq), with number of servings (srv) in parentheses when it differs from the other units. See note for quantity equivalents for foods in each group.[2] Oils are shown in grams (g).					
Fruits	1 c (2 srv)	1 c (2 srv)	1.5 c (3 srv)	1.5 c (3 srv)	1.5 c (3 srv)	2 c (4 srv)
Vegetables[3]	1 c (2 srv)	1.5 c (3 srv)	1.5 c (3 srv)	2 c (4 srv)	2.5 c (5 srv)	2.5 c (5 srv)
Dark green veg.	1 c/wk	1.5 c/wk	1.5 c/wk	2 c/wk	3 c/wk	3 c/wk
Orange veg.	0.5 c/wk	1 c/wk	1 c/wk	1.5 c/wk	2 c/wk	2 c/wk
Legumes	0.5 c/wk	1 c/wk	1 c/wk	2.5 c/wk	3 c/wk	3 c/wk
Starchy veg.	1.5 c/wk	2.5 c/wk	2.5 c/wk	2.5 c/wk	3 c/wk	3 c/wk
Other veg.	4 c/wk	4.5 c/wk	4.5 c/wk	5.5 c/wk	6.5 c/wk	6.5 c/wk
Grains[4]	3 oz-eq	4 oz-eq	5 oz-eq	5 oz-eq	6 oz-eq	6 oz-eq
Whole grains	1.5	2	2.5	3	3	3
Other grains	1.5	2	2.5	2	3	3
Lean meat and beans	2 oz-eq	3 oz-eq	4 oz-eq	5 oz-eq	5 oz-eq	5.5 oz-eq
Milk	2 c	2 c	2 c	3 c	3 c	3 c
Oils[5]	15 g	17 g	17 g	22 g	24 g	27 g
Discretionary calorie allowance[6]	165	171	171	132	195	267

Daily Amount of Food from Each Group (vegetable subgroup amounts are per week)

Calorie Level	2200	2400	2600	2800	3000	3200
Fruits	2 c	2 c	2 c	2.5 c	2.5 c	2.5 c
	(4 srv)	(4 srv)	(4 srv)	(5 srv)	(5 srv)	(5 srv)
Vegetables[3]	3 c	3 c	3.5 c	3.5 c	4 c	4 c
	(6 srv)	(6 srv)	(7 srv)	(7 srv)	(8 srv)	(8 srv)
Dark green veg.	3 c/wk	3 c/wk	3 c/wk	3 c/wk	3 c/wk	3 c/wk
Orange veg.	2 c/wk	2 c/wk	2.5 c/wk	2.5 c/wk	2.5 c/wk	2.5 c/wk
Legumes	3 c/wk	3 c/wk	3.5 c/wk	3.5 c/wk	3.5 c/wk	3.5 c/wk
Starchy veg.	6 c/wk	6 c/wk	7 c/wk	7 c/wk	9 c/wk	9 c/wk
Other veg.	7 c/wk	7 c/wk	8.5 c/wk	8.5 c/wk	10 c/wk	10 c/wk
Grains[4]	7 oz-eq	8 oz-eq	9 oz-eq	10 oz-eq	10 oz-eq	10 oz-eq
Whole grains	3.5	4	4.5	5	5	5
Other grains	3.5	4	4.5	5	5	5
Lean meat and beans	6 oz-eq	6.5 oz-eq	6.5 oz-eq	7 oz-eq	7 oz-eq	7 oz-eq
Milk	3 c	3 c	3 c	3 c	3 c	3 c
Oils[5]	29 g	31 g	34 g	36 g	44 g	51g
Discretionary calorie allowance[6]	290	362	410	426	512	648

[1] Food items included in each group and subgroup:

Fruits - All fresh, frozen, canned, and dried fruits and fruit juices, for example, oranges and orange juice, apples and apple juice, bananas, grapes, melons, berries, raisins. In developing the food patterns, only fruits and juices with no added sugars or fats were used. See note 6 on discretionary calories if products with added sugars or fats are consumed.

Vegetables - In developing the food patterns, only vegetables with no added fats or sugars were used. See note 6 on discretionary calories if products with added fats or sugars are consumed.

Dark green vegetables - All fresh, frozen, and canned dark green vegetables, cooked or raw: for example, broccoli; spinach; romaine; collard, turnip, and mustard greens.

Orange vegetables - All fresh, frozen, and canned orange and deep yellow vegetables, cooked or raw: for example, carrots, sweetpotatoes, winter squash, and pumpkin.

Legumes - All cooked dry beans and peas and soybean products: for example, pinto beans, kidney beans, lentils, chickpeas, tofu, (dry beans and peas). (See comment under meat and beans group about counting legumes in the vegetable or the meat and beans group.)

Starchy vegetables - All fresh, frozen, and canned starchy vegetables: for example, white potatoes, corn, green peas.

Grains - In developing the food patterns, only grains in low-fat and low-sugar forms were used. See note 6 on discretionary calories if products that are higher in fat and/or added sugars are consumed.

Whole grains - All whole-grain products and whole grains used as ingredients: for example, whole-wheat and rye breads, whole-grain cereals and crackers, oatmeal, and brown rice.

Other grains - All refined grain products and refined grains used as ingredients: for example, white breads, enriched grain cereals and crackers, enriched pasta, white rice. See note 6 on discretionary calories if higher fat products are consumed. Dry beans and peas and soybean products are considered part of this group as well as the vegetable group, but should be counted in one group only.

Milk, yogurt, and cheese (milk) - All milks, yogurts, frozen yogurts, dairy desserts, cheeses (except cream cheese), including lactose-free and lactose-reduced products. Most choices should be fat-free or low-fat. In developing the food patterns, only fat-free milk was used. See note 6 on discretionary calories if low-fat, reduced-fat, or whole milk or milk products or milk products that contain added sugars are consumed. Calcium-fortified soy beverages are an option for those who want a non-dairy calcium source.

[2] Quantity equivalents for each food group:

Grains - The following each count as 1 oz-equivalent (1 serving) of grains: ½ cup cooked rice, pasta, or cooked cereal; 1 oz dry pasta or rice; 1 slice bread; 1 small muffin (1 oz); 1 cup ready-to-eat cereal flakes.

Fruits and vegetables - The following each count as 1 cup (2 servings) of fruits or vegetables: 1 cup cut-up raw or cooked fruit or vegetable, 1 cup fruit or vegetable juice, 2 cups leafy salad greens.

Meat and beans - The following each count as 1 oz-equivalent: 1 oz lean meat, poultry, or fish; 1 egg; ¼ cup cooked dry beans or tofu; 1 tbsp peanut butter; ½ oz nuts or seeds.

Milk - The following each count as 1 cup (1 serving) of milk: 1 cup milk or yogurt, 1½ oz natural cheese such as cheddar cheese or 2 oz processed cheese. Discretionary calories must be counted for all choices, except fat-free milk.

[3] Explanation of vegetable subgroup amounts: Vegetable subgroup amounts are shown in this table as weekly amounts, because it would be difficult for consumers to select foods from each subgroup daily. A daily amount that is one-seventh of the weekly amount listed is used in calculations of nutrient and energy levels in each pattern.

[4] Explanation of grain subgroup amounts: The whole grain subgroup amounts shown in this table represent at least three 1-oz servings and one-half of the total amount as whole grains for all calorie levels of 1600 and above. This is the minimum suggested amount of whole grains to consume as part of the food patterns. More whole grains up to all of the grains recommended may be selected, with offsetting decreases in the amounts of other (enriched) grains. In patterns designed for younger children (1000, 1200, and 1400 calories), one-half of the total amount of grains is shown as whole grains.

[5] Explanation of oils: *Trans* fats shown in this table represent the amounts added to foods during processing, cooking, or at the table. Oils and soft margarines include vegetable oils and soft vegetable oil table spreads that have no *trans* fats. The amounts of oils listed in this table are not considered to be part of discretionary calories because they are a major source of the vitamin E and polyunsaturated fatty acids, including the essential fatty acids, in the food pattern. In contrast, solid fats are listed separately in the discretionary calorie table (Table C-3) because, compared with oils, they are higher in saturated fatty acids and lower in vitamin E and polyunsaturated and monounsaturated fatty acids, including essential fatty acids. The amounts of each type of fat in the food intake pattern were based on 60% oils and/or soft margarines with no *trans* fats and 40% solid fat. The amounts in typical American diets are about 42% oils or soft margarines and about 58% solid fats.

[6] Explanation of discretionary calorie allowance: The discretionary calorie allowance is the remaining amount of calories in each food pattern after selecting the specified number of nutrient-dense forms of foods in each food group. The number of discretionary calories assumes that food items in each food group are selected in nutrient-dense forms (that is, forms that are fat-free or low-fat and that contain no added sugars). Solid fat and sugar calories always need to be counted as discretionary calories, as in the following examples: The fat in low-fat, reduced fat, or whole milk or milk products or cheese and the sugar and fat in chocolate milk, ice cream, pudding, etc. The fat in higher fat meats (e.g., ground beef with more than 5% fat by weight, poultry with skin, higher fat luncheon meats, sausages). The sugars added to fruits and fruit juices with added sugars or fruits canned in syrup. The added fat and/or sugars in vegetables prepared with added fat or sugars. The added fats and/or sugars in grain products containing higher levels of fats and/or sugars (e.g., sweetened cereals, higher fat crackers, pies and other pastries, cakes, cookies).

Total discretionary calories should be limited to the amounts shown in the table at each calorie level. The number of discretionary calories is lower in the 1600-calorie pattern than in the 1000-, 1200-, and 1400-calorie patterns. These lower calorie patterns are designed to meet the nutrient needs of children 2 to 8 years. The nutrient goals for the 1600-calorie pattern are set to meet the needs of adult women, which are higher and require more calories used in selections from the basic food groups. Additional information about discretionary calories, including an example of the division of these calories between solid fats and added sugars, is provided in Table C-3.

Table C-3 Discretionary Calorie Allowance in the USDA Food Guide

The discretionary calorie allowance is the remaining amount of calories in each calorie level after nutrient-dense forms of foods in each food group are selected. This table shows the number of discretionary calories remaining in each calorie level if nutrient-dense foods are selected. Those trying to lose weight may choose not to use discretionary calories. For those wanting to maintain their weight, discretionary calories may be used to increase the amount of food selected from each food group; to consume foods that are not in the lowest fat form (such as 2% milk or medium-fat meat) or that contain added sugars; to add oil, fat, or sugars to foods; or to consume alcohol. The table shows an example of how these calories may be divided between solid fats and added sugars.

Discretionary calories that remain at each calorie level

Food Guide calorie level	1,000	1,200	1,400	1,600	1,800	2,000	2,200	2,400	2,600	2,800	3,000	3,200
Discretionary calories[1]	165	171	171	132	195	267	290	362	410	426	512	648

Example of division of discretionary calories: Solid fats are shown in grams (g); added sugars in grams (g) and teaspoons (tsp).

Solid fats[2]	11 g	14 g	14 g	11 g	15 g	18 g	19 g	22 g	24 g	24 g	29 g	34 g
Added sugars[3]	20 g (5 tsp)	16 g (4 tsp)	16 g (4 tsp)	12 g (3 tsp)	20 g (5 tsp)	32 g (8 tsp)	36 g (9 tsp)	48 g (12 tsp)	56 g (14 tsp)	60 g (15 tsp)	72g (18 tsp)	96 g (24 tsp)

[1] Discretionary calories: In developing the Food Guide, food items in nutrient-dense forms (that is, forms that are fat-free or low-fat and that contain no added sugars) were used. The number of discretionary calories assumes that food items in each food group are selected in nutrient-dense forms. Solid fat and sugar calories always need to be counted as discretionary calories, as in the following examples: The fat in low-fat, reduced fat, or whole milk or milk products or cheese and the sugar and fat in chocolate milk, ice cream, pudding, etc. The fat in higher fat meats (e.g., ground beef with more than 5% fat by weight, poultry with skin, higher fat luncheon meats, sausages). The sugars added to fruits and fruit juices with added sugars or fruits canned in syrup. The added fat and/or sugars in vegetables prepared with added fat or sugars. The added fats and/or sugars in grain products containing higher levels of fats and/or sugars (e.g., sweetened cereals, higher fat crackers, pies and other pastries, cakes, cookies).

Total discretionary calories should be limited to the amounts shown in the table at each calorie level. The number of discretionary calories is lower in the 1600-calorie pattern than in the 1000-, 1200-, and 1400-calorie patterns. These lower calorie patterns are designed to meet the nutrient needs of children 2 to 8 years. The nutrient goals for the 1600-calorie pattern are set to meet the needs of adult women, which are higher and require more calories used in selections from the basic food groups. The calories assigned to discretionary calories may be used to increase intake from the basic food groups; to select foods from these groups that are higher in fat or with added sugars; to add oils, solid fats, or sugars to foods or beverages; or to consume alcohol. See note 2 on limits for solid fats.

[2] Solid fats: Amounts of solid fats listed in the table represent about 7–8% of calories from saturated fat. Foods in each food group are represented in their lowest fat forms, such as fat-free milk and skinless chicken. Solid fats shown in this table represent the amounts of fats that may be added in cooking or at the table, and fats consumed when higher fat items are selected from the food groups (e.g., whole milk instead of fat-free milk, chicken with skin, or cookies instead of bread), without exceeding the recommended limits on saturated fat intake. Solid fats include meat and poultry fats eaten either as part of the meat or poultry product or separately; milk fat such as that in whole milk, cheese, and butter; shortenings used in baked products; and hard margarines.

Solid fats and oils are separated because their fatty acid compositions differ. Solid fats are higher in saturated fatty acids, and commonly consumed oils and soft margarines with no *trans* fats are higher in vitamin E and polyunsaturated and monounsaturated fatty acids, including essential fatty acids.

The gram weights for solid fats are the amounts of these products that can be included in the pattern and are not identical to the amount of lipids in these items, because some products (margarines, butter) contain water or other ingredients, in addition to lipids.

[3] Added sugars: Added sugars are the sugars and syrups added to foods and beverages in processing or preparation, not the naturally occurring sugars in fruits or milk. The amounts of added sugars suggested in the example are **not** specific recommendations for amounts of added sugars to consume, but rather represent the amounts that can be included at each calorie level without over-consuming calories. The suggested amounts of added sugars may be helpful as part of the Food Guide to allow for some sweetened foods or beverages, without exceeding energy needs. This use of added sugars as a calorie balance requires two assumptions: (1) that selections are made from all food groups in accordance with the suggested amounts, and (2) that additional fats are used in the amounts shown, which, together with the fats in the core food groups, represent about 27–30% of calories from fat.

Appendix D
Food Sources of
Selected Nutrients

Table D-1 Food Sources of Potassium

Sources of potassium ranked by milligrams of potassium per standard amount, also showing calories in the standard amount. (The AI for adults is 4700 mg/day potassium.)

Food, Standard Amount	Potassium (mg)	Calories
Sweet potato, baked, 1 potato (146 g)	694	131
Tomato paste, ¼ cup	664	54
Beet greens, cooked, ½ cup	655	19
Potato, baked, flesh, 1 potato (156 g)	610	145
White beans, canned, ½ cup	595	153
Yogurt, plain, non-fat, 8-oz container	579	127
Tomato puree, ½ cup	549	48
Clams, canned, 3 oz	534	126
Yogurt, plain, low-fat, 8-oz container	531	143
Prune juice, ¾ cup	530	136
Carrot juice, ¾ cup	517	71
Blackstrap molasses, 1 tbsp	498	47
Halibut, cooked, 3 oz	490	119
Soybeans, green, cooked, ½ cup	485	127
Tuna, yellowfin, cooked, 3 oz	484	118
Lima beans, cooked, ½ cup	484	104
Winter squash, cooked, ½ cup	448	40
Soybeans, mature, cooked, ½ cup	443	149
Rockfish, Pacific, cooked, 3 oz	442	103
Cod, Pacific, cooked, 3 oz	439	89
Bananas, 1 medium	422	105
Spinach, cooked, ½ cup	419	21
Tomato juice, ¾ cup	417	31
Tomato sauce, ½ cup	405	39
Peaches, dried, uncooked, ¼ cup	398	96
Prunes, stewed, ½ cup	398	133
Milk, non-fat, 1 cup	382	83
Pork chop, center loin, cooked, 3 oz	382	197
Apricots, dried, uncooked, ¼ cup	378	78
Rainbow trout, farmed, cooked, 3 oz	375	144
Pork loin, center rib (roasts), lean, roasted, 3 oz	371	190

Food, Standard Amount	Potassium (mg)	Calories
Buttermilk, cultured, low-fat, 1 cup	370	98
Cantaloupe, ¼ medium	368	47
1–2% milk, 1 cup	366	102–122
Honeydew melon, ⅛ medium	365	58
Lentils, cooked, ½ cup	365	115
Plantains, cooked, ½ cup slices	358	90
Kidney beans, cooked, ½ cup	358	112
Orange juice, ¾ cup	355	85
Split peas, cooked, ½ cup	355	116
Yogurt, plain, whole milk, 8-oz container	352	138

Nutrient values from Agricultural Research Service (ARS), *Nutrient Database for Standard Reference,* Release 17. Foods from ARS single nutrient reports, sorted in descending order by nutrient content in terms of common household measures. Food items and weights in the single nutrient reports adapted from those in the 2002 revision of USDA Home and Garden Bulletin No. 72, *Nutritive Value of Foods.* Mixed dishes and multiple preparations of the same food item have been omitted from this table.

Table D-2 Food Sources of Vitamin E

Food sources of vitamin E ranked by milligrams of vitamin E per standard amount; also calories in the standard amount. (All provide ≥ 10% of RDA for vitamin E for adults, which is 15 mg α-tocopherol [AT]/day.)

Food, Standard Amount	AT (mg)	Calories
Fortified ready-to-eat cereals, ~1 oz	1.6–12.8	90–107
Sunflower seeds, dry roasted, 1 oz	7.4	165
Almonds, 1 oz	7.3	164
Sunflower oil, high linoleic, 1 tbsp	5.6	120
Cottonseed oil, 1 tbsp	4.8	120
Safflower oil, high oleic, 1 tbsp	4.6	120
Hazelnuts (filberts), 1 oz	4.3	178
Mixed nuts, dry roasted, 1 oz	3.1	168
Turnip greens, frozen, cooked, ½ cup	2.9	24
Tomato paste, ¼ cup	2.8	54
Pine nuts, 1 oz	2.6	191
Peanut butter, 2 tbsp	2.5	192
Tomato puree, ½ cup	2.5	48
Tomato sauce, ½ cup	2.5	39
Canola oil, 1 tbsp	2.4	124
Wheat germ, toasted, plain, 2 tbsp	2.3	54
Peanuts, 1 oz	2.2	166
Avocado, raw, ½ avocado	2.1	161
Carrot juice, canned, ¾ cup	2.1	71
Peanut oil, 1 tbsp	2.1	119
Corn oil, 1 tbsp	1.9	120
Olive oil, 1 tbsp	1.9	119
Spinach, cooked, ½ cup	1.9	21
Dandelion greens, cooked, ½ cup	1.8	18
Sardine, Atlantic, in oil, drained, 3 oz	1.7	177
Blue crab, cooked/canned, 3 oz	1.6	84
Brazil nuts, 1 oz	1.6	186
Herring, Atlantic, pickled, 3 oz	1.5	222

Nutrient values from Agricultural Research Service (ARS), *Nutrient Database for Standard Reference,* Release 17. Foods from ARS single nutrient reports, sorted in descending order by nutrient content in terms of common household measures. Food items and weights in the single nutrient reports adapted from those in the 2002 revision of USDA Home and Garden Bulletin No. 72, *Nutritive Value of Foods.* Mixed dishes and multiple preparations of the same food item have been omitted from this table.

Table D-3 Food Sources of Iron

Food sources of iron ranked by milligrams of iron per standard amount; also calories in the standard amount. (All are ≥ 10% of RDA for teen and adult females, which is 18 mg/day.)

Food, Standard Amount	Iron (mg)	Calories
Clams, canned, drained, 3 oz	23.8	126
Fortified ready-to-eat cereals (various), ~ 1 oz	1.8–21.1	54–127
Oysters, eastern, wild, cooked, moist heat, 3 oz	10.2	116
Organ meats (liver, giblets), various, cooked, 3 oz[a]	5.2-9.9	134-235
Fortified instant cooked cereals (various), 1 packet	4.9-8.1	Varies
Soybeans, mature, cooked, ½ cup	4.4	149
Pumpkin and squash seed kernels, roasted, 1 oz	4.2	148
White beans, canned, ½ cup	3.9	153
Blackstrap molasses, 1 tbsp	3.5	47
Lentils, cooked, ½ cup	3.3	115
Spinach, cooked from fresh, ½ cup	3.2	21
Beef, chuck, blade roast, lean, cooked, 3 oz	3.1	215
Beef, bottom round, lean, 0" fat, all grades, cooked, 3 oz	2.8	182
Kidney beans, cooked, ½ cup	2.6	112
Sardines, canned in oil, drained, 3 oz	2.5	177
Beef, rib, lean, ¼" fat, all grades, 3 oz	2.4	195
Chickpeas, cooked, ½ cup	2.4	134
Duck, meat only, roasted, 3 oz	2.3	171
Lamb, shoulder, arm, lean, ¼" fat, choice, cooked, 3 oz	2.3	237
Prune juice, ¾ cup	2.3	136
Shrimp, canned, 3 oz	2.3	102
Cowpeas, cooked, ½ cup	2.2	100
Ground beef, 15% fat, cooked, 3 oz	2.2	212
Tomato puree, ½ cup	2.2	48
Lima beans, cooked, ½ cup	2.2	108
Soybeans, green, cooked, ½ cup	2.2	127
Navy beans, cooked, ½ cup	2.1	127
Refried beans, ½ cup	2.1	118
Beef, top sirloin, lean, 0" fat, all grades, cooked, 3 oz	2.0	156
Tomato paste, ¼ cup	2.0	54

[a] High in cholesterol.

Nutrient values from Agricultural Research Service (ARS). *Nutrient Database for Standard Reference*, Release 17. Foods from ARS single nutrient reports, sorted in descending order by nutrient content in terms of common household measures. Food items and weights in the single nutrient reports adapted from those in the 2002 revision of USDA Home and Garden Bulletin No. 72, *Nutritive Value of Foods*. Mixed dishes and multiple preparations of the same food item have been omitted from this table.

Table D-4 Nondairy Food Sources of Calcium

Nondairy food sources of calcium are ranked by milligrams of calcium per standard amount; also calories in the standard amount. The bioavailability may vary. (The AI for adults is 1000 mg/day.)[a]

Food, Standard Amount	Calcium (mg)	Calories
Fortified ready-to-eat cereals (various), 1 oz	236–1043	88–106
Soy beverage, calcium fortified, 1 cup	368	98
Sardines, Atlantic, in oil, drained, 3 oz	325	177
Tofu, firm, prepared with nigari,[b] ½ cup	253	88
Pink salmon, canned, with bone, 3 oz	181	118
Collards, cooked from frozen, ½ cup	178	31
Molasses, blackstrap, 1 tbsp	172	47
Spinach, cooked from frozen, ½ cup	146	30
Soybeans, green, cooked, ½ cup	130	127
Turnip greens, cooked from frozen, ½ cup	124	24
Ocean perch, Atlantic, cooked, 3 oz	116	103
Oatmeal, plain and flavored, instant, fortified, 1 packet prepared	99–110	97–157
Cowpeas, cooked, ½ cup	106	80
White beans, canned, ½ cup	96	153
Kale, cooked from frozen, ½ cup	90	20
Okra, cooked from frozen, ½ cup	88	26
Soybeans, mature, cooked, ½ cup	88	149
Blue crab, canned, 3 oz	86	84
Beet greens, cooked from fresh, ½ cup	82	19
Pak-choi, Chinese cabbage, cooked from fresh, ½ cup	79	10
Clams, canned, 3 oz	78	126
Dandelion greens, cooked from fresh, ½ cup	74	17
Rainbow trout, farmed, cooked, 3 oz	73	144

[a] Both calcium content and bioavailability should be considered when selecting dietary sources of calcium. Some plant foods have calcium that is well absorbed, but the large quantity of plant foods that would be needed to provide as much calcium as in a glass of milk may be unachievable for many. Many other calcium-fortified foods are available, but the percentage of calcium that can be absorbed is unavailable for many of them.
[b] Calcium sulfate and magnesium chloride.
Nutrient values from Agricultural Research Service (ARS). *Nutrient Database for Standard Reference*, Release 17. Foods from ARS single nutrient reports, sorted in descending order by nutrient content in terms of common household measures. Food items and weights in the single nutrient reports adapted from those in the 2002 revision of USDA Home and Garden Bulletin No. 72, *Nutritive Value of Foods*. Mixed dishes and multiple preparations of the same food item have been omitted from this table.

Table D-5 Food Sources of Calcium

Food sources of calcium ranked by milligrams of calcium per standard amount; also calories in the standard amount. (All are ≥ 20% of AI for adults 19–50, which is 1000 mg/day.)

Food, Standard Amount	Calcium (mg)	Calories
Plain yogurt, non-fat (13 g protein/8 oz), 8-oz container	452	127
Romano cheese, 1.5 oz	452	165
Pasteurized process Swiss cheese, 2 oz	438	190
Plain yogurt, low-fat (12 g protein/8 oz), 8-oz container	415	143
Fruit yogurt, low-fat (10 g protein/8 oz), 8-oz container	345	232
Swiss cheese, 1.5 oz	336	162
Ricotta cheese, part skim, ½ cup	335	170
Pasteurized process American cheese food, 2 oz	323	188
Provolone cheese, 1.5 oz	321	150
Mozzarella cheese, part-skim, 1.5 oz	311	129
Cheddar cheese, 1.5 oz	307	171
Fat-free (skim) milk, 1 cup	306	83
Muenster cheese, 1.5 oz	305	156
1% low-fat milk, 1 cup	290	102
Low-fat chocolate milk (1%), 1 cup	288	158
2% reduced fat milk, 1 cup	285	122
Reduced fat chocolate milk (2%), 1 cup	285	180
Buttermilk, low-fat, 1 cup	284	98
Chocolate milk, 1 cup	280	208
Whole milk, 1 cup	276	146
Yogurt, plain, whole milk (8 g protein/8 oz), 8-oz container	275	138
Ricotta cheese, whole milk, ½ cup	255	214
Blue cheese, 1.5 oz	225	150
Mozzarella cheese, whole milk, 1.5 oz	215	128
Feta cheese, 1.5 oz	210	113

Nutrient values from Agricultural Research Service (ARS). *Nutrient Database for Standard Reference*, Release 17. Foods from ARS single nutrient reports, sorted in descending order by nutrient content in terms of common household measures. Food items and weights in the single nutrient reports adapted from those in the 2002 revision of USDA Home and Garden Bulletin No. 72, *Nutritive Value of Foods*. Mixed dishes and multiple preparations of the same food item have been omitted from this table.

Table D-6 Food Sources of Vitamin A

Food sources of vitamin A ranked by micrograms Retinol Activity Equivalents (RAE) of vitamin A per standard amount; also calories in the standard amount. (All are ≥ 20% of RDA for adult men, which is 900 mcg/day RAE.)

Food, Standard Amount	Vitamin A (mcg RAE)	Calories
Organ meats (liver, giblets), various, cooked, 3 oz[a]	1490–9126	134–235
Carrot juice, ¾ cup	1692	71
Sweet potato with peel, baked, 1 medium	1096	103
Pumpkin, canned, ½ cup	953	42
Carrots, cooked from fresh, ½ cup	671	27
Spinach, cooked from frozen, ½ cup	573	30
Collards, cooked from frozen, ½ cup	489	31
Kale, cooked from frozen, ½ cup	478	20
Mixed vegetables, canned, ½ cup	474	40
Turnip greens, cooked from frozen, ½ cup	441	24
Instant cooked cereals, fortified, prepared, 1 packet	285–376	75–97
Various ready-to-eat cereals, with added vitamin A, ~1 oz	180–376	100–117
Carrot, raw, 1 small	301	20
Beet greens, cooked, ½ cup	276	19
Winter squash, cooked, ½ cup	268	38
Dandelion greens, cooked, ½ cup	260	18
Cantaloupe, raw, ¼ medium melon	233	46
Mustard greens, cooked, ½ cup	221	11
Pickled herring, 3 oz	219	222
Red sweet pepper, cooked, ½ cup	186	19
Chinese cabbage, cooked, ½ cup	180	10

[a] High in cholesterol.

Nutrient values from Agricultural Research Service (ARS). *Nutrient Database for Standard Reference,* Release 17. Foods from ARS single nutrient reports, sorted in descending order by nutrient content in terms of common household measures. Food items and weights in the single nutrient reports adapted from those in the 2002 revision of USDA Home and Garden Bulletin No. 72, *Nutritive Value of Foods.* Mixed dishes and multiple preparations of the same food item have been omitted from this table.

Table D-7 Food Sources of Magnesium

Food sources of magnesium ranked by milligrams of magnesium per standard amount; also calories in the standard amount. (All are ≥ 10% of RDA for adult men, which is 420 mg/day.)

Food, Standard Amount	Magnesium (mg)	Calories
Pumpkin and squash seed kernels, roasted, 1 oz	151	148
Brazil nuts, 1 oz	107	186
Bran ready-to-eat cereal (100%), ~1 oz	103	74
Halibut, cooked, 3 oz	91	119
Quinoa, dry, ¼ cup	89	159
Spinach, canned, ½ cup	81	25
Almonds, 1 oz	78	164
Spinach, cooked from fresh, ½ cup	78	20
Buckwheat flour, ¼ cup	75	101
Cashews, dry roasted, 1 oz	74	163
Soybeans, mature, cooked, ½ cup	74	149
Pine nuts, dried, 1 oz	71	191
Mixed nuts, oil roasted, with peanuts, 1 oz	67	175
White beans, canned, ½ cup	67	154
Pollock, walleye, cooked, 3 oz	62	96
Black beans, cooked, ½ cup	60	114
Bulgur, dry, ¼ cup	57	120
Oat bran, raw, ¼ cup	55	58
Soybeans, green, cooked, ½ cup	54	127
Tuna, yellowfin, cooked, 3 oz	54	118
Artichokes (hearts), cooked, ½ cup	50	42
Peanuts, dry roasted, 1 oz	50	166
Lima beans, baby, cooked from frozen, ½ cup	50	95
Beet greens, cooked, ½ cup	49	19
Navy beans, cooked, ½ cup	48	127
Tofu, firm, prepared with nigari, ½ cup	47	88
Okra, cooked from frozen, ½ cup	47	26
Soy beverage, 1 cup	47	127
Cowpeas, cooked, ½ cup	46	100
Hazelnuts, 1 oz	46	178

Food, Standard Amount	Magnesium (mg)	Calories
Oat bran muffin, 1 oz	45	77
Great northern beans, cooked, ½ cup	44	104
Oat bran, cooked, ½ cup	44	44
Buckwheat groats, roasted, cooked, ½ cup	43	78
Brown rice, cooked, ½ cup	42	108
Haddock, cooked, 3 oz	42	95

[a] Calcium sulfate and magnesium chloride.

Nutrient values from Agricultural Research Service (ARS). *Nutrient Database for Standard Reference,* Release 17. Foods from ARS single nutrient reports, sorted in descending order by nutrient content in terms of common household measures. Food items and weights in the single nutrient reports adapted from those in the 2002 revision of USDA Home and Garden Bulletin No. 72, *Nutritive Value of Foods.* Mixed dishes and multiple preparations of the same food item have been omitted from this table.

Table D-8 Food Sources of Dietary Fiber

Food sources of dietary fiber ranked by grams of dietary fiber per standard amount; also calories in the standard amount. (All are ≥ 10% of AI for adult women, which is 25 g/day.)

Food, Standard Amount	Dietary Fiber (g)	Calories
Navy beans, cooked, ½ cup	9.5	128
Bran ready-to-eat cereal (100%), ½ cup	8.8	78
Kidney beans, canned, ½ cup	8.2	109
Split peas, cooked, ½ cup	8.1	116
Lentils, cooked, ½ cup	7.8	115
Black beans, cooked, ½ cup	7.5	114
Pinto beans, cooked, ½ cup	7.7	122
Lima beans, cooked, ½ cup	6.6	108
Artichoke, globe, cooked, 1 each	6.5	60
White beans, canned, ½ cup	6.3	154
Chickpeas, cooked, ½ cup	6.2	135
Great northern beans, cooked, ½ cup	6.2	105
Cowpeas, cooked, ½ cup	5.6	100
Soybeans, mature, cooked, ½ cup	5.2	149
Bran ready-to-eat cereals, various, ~1 oz	2.6–5.0	90–108
Crackers, rye wafers, plain, 2 wafers	5.0	74
Sweet potato, baked, with peel, 1 medium (146 g)	4.8	131
Asian pear, raw, 1 small	4.4	51
Green peas, cooked, ½ cup	4.4	67
Whole-wheat English muffin, 1 each	4.4	134
Pear, raw, 1 small	4.3	81
Bulgur, cooked, ½ cup	4.1	76
Mixed vegetables, cooked, ½ cup	4.0	59
Raspberries, raw, ½ cup	4.0	32
Sweet potato, boiled, no peel, 1 medium (156 g)	3.9	119
Blackberries, raw, ½ cup	3.8	31
Potato, baked, with skin, 1 medium	3.8	161
Soybeans, green, cooked, ½ cup	3.8	127
Stewed prunes, ½ cup	3.8	133
Figs, dried, ¼ cup	3.7	93

Table D-8 (continued)

Food, Standard Amount	Dietary Fiber (g)	Calories
Dates, ¼ cup	3.6	126
Oat bran, raw, ¼ cup	3.6	58
Pumpkin, canned, ½ cup	3.6	42
Spinach, frozen, cooked, ½ cup	3.5	30
Shredded wheat ready-to-eat cereals, various, ~1 oz	2.8–3.4	96
Almonds, 1 oz	3.3	164
Apple with skin, raw, 1 medium	3.3	72
Brussels sprouts, frozen, cooked, ½ cup	3.2	33
Whole-wheat spaghetti, cooked, ½ cup	3.1	87
Banana, 1 medium	3.1	105
Orange, raw, 1 medium	3.1	62
Oat bran muffin, 1 small	3.0	178
Guava, 1 medium	3.0	37
Pearled barley, cooked, ½ cup	3.0	97
Sauerkraut, canned, solids, and liquids, ½ cup	3.0	23
Tomato paste, ¼ cup	2.9	54
Winter squash, cooked, ½ cup	2.9	38
Broccoli, cooked, ½ cup	2.8	26
Parsnips, cooked, chopped, ½ cup	2.8	55
Turnip greens, cooked, ½ cup	2.5	15
Collards, cooked, ½ cup	2.7	25
Okra, frozen, cooked, ½ cup	2.6	26
Peas, edible-podded, cooked, ½ cup	2.5	42

Nutrient values from USDA Agricultural Research Service (http://www.ARS.USDA.gov/main/min.htm). ARS *Nutrient Database for Standard Reference,* Release 17. Foods from single nutrient reports, which are sorted either by food description or in descending order by nutrient content in terms of common household measures. The food items and weights in these reports adapted from those in the 2002 revision of USDA Home and Garden Bulletin No. 72, *Nutritive Value of Foods.* Mixed dishes and multiple preparations of the same food item have been omitted.

Table D-9 Food Sources of Vitamin C

Food sources of vitamin C ranked by milligrams of vitamin C per standard amount; also calories in the standard amount. (All provide ≥ 20% of RDA for adult men, which is 90 mg/day.)

Food, Standard Amount	Vitamin C (mg)	Calories
Guava, raw, ½ cup	188	56
Red sweet pepper, raw, ½ cup	142	20
Red sweet pepper, cooked, ½ cup	116	19
Kiwi fruit, 1 medium	70	46
Orange, raw, 1 medium	70	62
Orange juice, ¾ cup	61–93	79–84
Green pepper, sweet, raw, ½ cup	60	15
Green pepper, sweet, cooked, ½ cup	51	19
Grapefruit juice, ¾ cup	50–70	71–86
Vegetable juice cocktail, ¾ cup	50	34
Strawberries, raw, ½ cup	49	27
Brussels sprouts, cooked, ½ cup	48	28
Cantaloupe, ¼ medium	47	51
Papaya, raw, ¼ medium	47	30
Kohlrabi, cooked, ½ cup	45	24
Broccoli, raw, ½ cup	39	15
Edible pod peas, cooked, ½ cup	38	34
Broccoli, cooked, ½ cup	37	26
Sweetpotato, canned, ½ cup	34	116
Tomato juice, ¾ cup	33	31
Cauliflower, cooked, ½ cup	28	17
Pineapple, raw, ½ cup	28	37
Kale, cooked, ½ cup	27	18
Mango, ½ cup	23	54

Nutrient values from Agricultural Research Service (ARS). *Nutrient Database for Standard Reference,* Release 17. Foods from ARS single nutrient reports, sorted in descending order by nutrient content in terms of common household measures. Food items and weights in the single nutrient reports adapted from those in the 2002 revision of USDA Home and Garden Bulletin No. 72, *Nutritive Value of Foods.* Mixed dishes and multiple preparations of the same food item have been omitted from this table.

From *USDA Dietary Guidelines for Americans 2005,* Appendix B: Food Sources of Selected Nutrients. http://www.health.gov/dietaryguidelines/dga2005/document/html/appendixB.htm

Appendix E
Body Mass Index (BMI) for Children and Teens

BMI IS USED DIFFERENTLY WITH CHILDREN THAN IT IS WITH ADULTS

In children and teens, body mass index is used to assess underweight, overweight, and risk for overweight. Children's body fatness changes over the years as they grow. Also, girls and boys differ in their body fatness as they mature. This is why BMI for children, also referred to as BMI-for-age, is gender and age specific. BMI-for-age is plotted on gender-specific growth charts (see Figures E-1 to E-4). These charts are used for children and teens 2–20 years. For the 2000 CDC Growth Charts and additional information, visit CDC's National Center for Health Statistics at http://www.cdc.gov/growthcharts/.

Each of the CDC BMI-for-age gender-specific charts contains a series of curved lines indicating specific percentiles. Healthcare professionals use the established percentile cutoff points shown in the table to identify underweight and overweight in children.

Underweight	BMI-for-age < 5th percentile
Normal	BMI-for-age 5th percentile to < 85th percentile
At risk of overweight	BMI-for-age 85th percentile to < 95th percentile
Overweight	BMI-for-age > 95th percentile

SOURCES

Hammer, L. D., Kraemer, H. C., Wilson, D. M., Ritter, P. L., Dornbusch, S. M. Standardized percentile curves of body-mass index for children and adolescents. (1991) *American Journal of Disease of Children,* 145,259–263.

Pietrobelli, A., Faith, M. S., Allison, D. B., Gallagher, D., Chiumello, G., Heymsfield, S.B. Body mass index as a measure of adiposity among children and adolescents: A validation study. (1998) *Journal of Pediatrics,* 132,204–210.

Figure E-1 Length-for-Age and Weight-for-Age Percentiles: Birth to 36 Months: Boys.

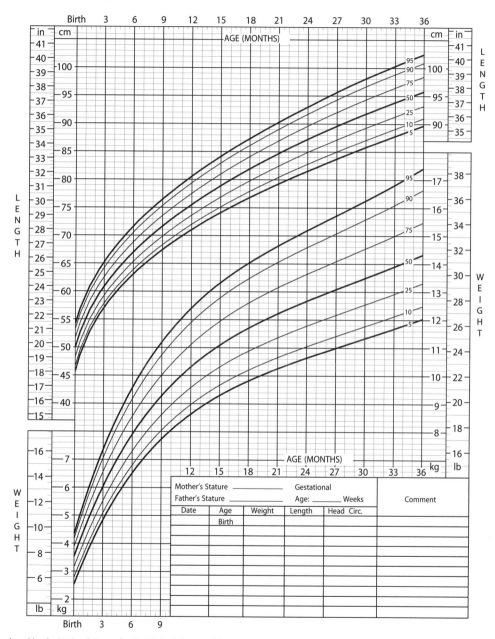

Developed by the National Center for Health Statistics in collaboration with the National Center for Chronic Disease Prevention and Health Promotion (2000).

Figure E-2 Length-for-Age and Weight-for-Age Percentiles: Birth to 36 Months: Girls.

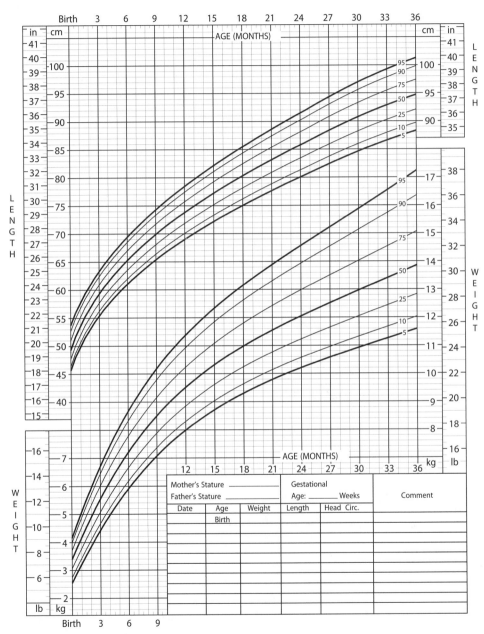

Developed by the National Center for Health Statistics in collaboration with the National Center for Chronic Disease Prevention and Health Promotion (2000).

Figure E-3 Body Mass Index-for-Age Percentiles: 2 to 20 Years: Boys.

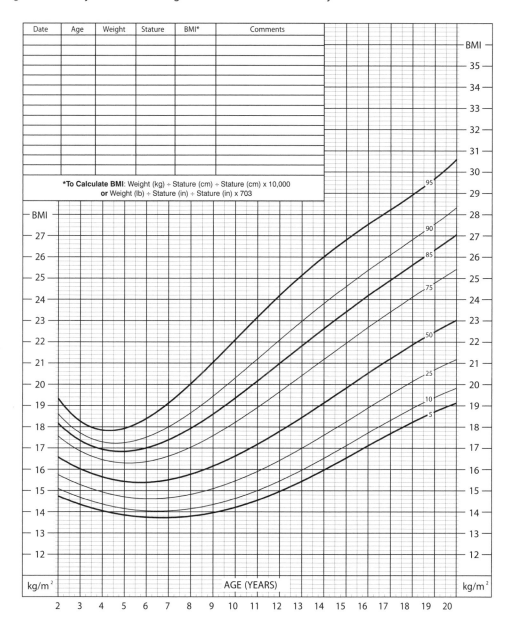

Date	Age	Weight	Stature	BMI*	Comments

*To Calculate BMI: Weight (kg) ÷ Stature (cm) ÷ Stature (cm) x 10,000
or Weight (lb) ÷ Stature (in) ÷ Stature (in) x 703

Developed by the National Center for Health Statistics in collaboration with the National Center for Chronic Disease Prevention and Health Promotion (2000).

Figure E-4 Body Mass Index-for-Age Percentiles: 2 to 20 Years: Girls.

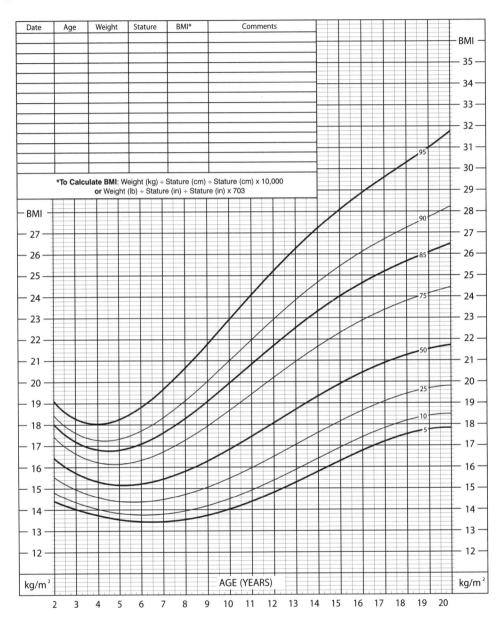

Date	Age	Weight	Stature	BMI*	Comments

*To Calculate BMI: Weight (kg) ÷ Stature (cm) ÷ Stature (cm) x 10,000
or Weight (lb) ÷ Stature (in) ÷ Stature (in) x 703

Developed by the National Center for Health Statistics in collaboration with the National Center for Chronic Disease Prevention and Health Promotion (2000).

Appendix F

MyPyramid Food Intake Pattern Calorie Levels

Table F-1 MyPyramid Food Intake Pattern Calorie Levels

MyPyramid assigns individuals to a calorie level based on that person's sex, age, and activity level. The chart identifies the calorie levels for males and females by age and activity level. Calorie levels are provided for each year of childhood, from 2–18 years, and for adults in 5-year increments.

Males				Females			
Activity level	**Sedentary***	**Mod. active***	**Active***	**Activity level**	**Sedentary***	**Mod. active***	**Active***
AGE				**AGE**			
2	1000	1000	1000	2	1000	1000	1000
3	1000	1400	1400	3	1000	1200	1400
4	1200	1400	1600	4	1200	1400	1400
5	1200	1400	1600	5	1200	1400	1600
6	1400	1600	1800	6	1200	1400	1600
7	1400	1600	1800	7	1200	1600	1800
8	1400	1600	2000	8	1400	1600	1800
9	1600	1800	2000	9	1400	1600	1800
10	1600	1800	2200	10	1400	1800	2000
11	1800	2000	2200	11	1600	1800	2000
12	1800	2200	2400	12	1600	2000	2200
13	2000	2200	2600	13	1600	2000	2200
14	2000	2400	2800	14	1800	2000	2400
15	2200	2600	3000	15	1800	2000	2400
16	2400	2800	3200	16	1800	2000	2400
17	2400	2800	3200	17	1800	2000	2400
18	2400	2800	3200	18	1800	2000	2400
19–20	2600	2800	3000	19–20	2000	2200	2400
21–25	2400	2800	3000	21–25	2000	2200	2400
26–30	2400	2600	3000	26–30	1800	2000	2400
31–35	2400	2600	3000	31–35	1800	2000	2200
36–40	2400	2600	2800	36–40	1800	2000	2200
41–45	2200	2600	2800	41–45	1800	2000	2200
46–50	2200	2400	2800	46–50	1800	2000	2200
51–55	2200	2400	2800	51–55	1600	1800	2200
56–60	2200	2400	2600	56–60	1600	1800	2200
61–65	2000	2400	2600	61–65	1600	1800	2000
66–70	2000	2200	2600	66–70	1600	1800	2000
71–75	2000	2200	2600	71–75	1600	1800	2000
76 and up	2000	2000	2400	76 and up	1600	1800	2000

*Calorie levels are based on the Estimated Energy Requirements (EER) and activity levels from the Institute of Medicine Dietary Reference Intakes Macronutrients Report, 2002. Sedentary = up to 30 minutes a day of moderate physical activity, in addition to daily activities. Mod. Active = 30–60 minutes a day of moderate physical activity, in addition to daily activities. Active = 60 minutes or more a day of moderate physical activity, in addition to daily activities.

USDA Center for Nutrition Policy and Promotion, April 2005. http://www.mypyramid.gov/professionals/pdf_calorie_levels.html

Appendix G

Remembering Sizes: Tips for Staying on Target!

Serving Sizes vs. Portion Sizes: What's the Difference?

Serving—A *standard* amount of food based on the Food Guide Pyramid, to give advice about how much to eat or to identify how many calories/nutrients are in a food.

Portion—The amount of food a person *chooses* to eat or is served. There is no standard portion size.

Common Foods: Typical portions vs. Recommended servings:

Meat, Poultry, Fish, Beans, Eggs, Nuts Group (2–3 servings daily) 5–7 ounces total

Common Foods	Typical Portion	Pyramid Servings in This Portion	Recommended Pyramid Serving Size
Steak	13 oz.	5	2–3 oz.
Scrambled Eggs	3 eggs	3	1 egg
Tuna Salad (in sandwich)	6 oz.	2	2–3 oz.

Breads, Cereal, Rice, and Pasta Group (6–11 servings daily)

Common Foods	Typical Portion	Pyramid Servings in This Portion	Recommended Pyramid Serving Size
Hamburger Bun	1 bun	2	½ bun
Medium Muffin	6 oz.	3	2 oz.
Bagel	4 oz.	4	1 oz.
Spaghetti	3 ½ cups (cooked)	7	½ cup (cooked)

Vegetable Group (3–5 servings daily) and Fruit Group (2–4 servings)

Common Foods	Typical Portion	Pyramid Servings in This Portion	Recommended Pyramid Serving Size
Orange Juice	1 large (12–16 oz.)	2–3	6 oz. (¾ cup)
Baked Potato	1 large (7 oz.)	3	1 small (2 ¼ oz.)

Fats and Sweets ("USE SPARINGLY")

Common Foods	Typical Portion	USDA Servings in This Portion	USDA Serving Size
Cream Cheese (on Bagel)	4 Tablespoons (2 oz.)	2	2 TB (1 oz.)
Soda (bottled)	20 oz.	2 ½	8 oz.
Salad Dressing	4 TB (2 oz.)	2	2 TB (1 oz.)

Inova Healthsource.

Remembering Serving Sizes: Tips for Staying on Target!

Using Items around the house:

 4 die   1 oz of cheese

 1 deck of playing cards   3 oz cooked meat

 1 golf ball   2 tbsp

 a computer mouse   1 small baked potato

 a baseball   1 cup

Using parts of your body:

 2 thumbs   1 ounce or 2 tbsp

 Palm of woman's hand   3 oz

 1 fist   1 cup

Inova Healthsource.

Glossary and References

GLOSSARY

Acceptable Macronutrient Distribution Ranges (AMDR)—Range of intake for a particular energy source associated with reduced risk of chronic disease, while providing intakes of essential nutrients. If an individual consumes in excess of the AMDR, there is a potential of increasing the risk of chronic diseases and/or insufficient intakes of essential nutrients.

Added Sugars—Sugars and syrups added to foods during processing or preparation. Added sugars do not include naturally occurring sugars such as those that occur in milk and fruits.

Adequate Intakes (AIs)—A recommended average daily nutrient intake level based on observed or experimentally determined approximations or estimates of mean nutrient intake by a group (or groups) of apparently healthy people. The AI is used when the Estimated Average Requirement cannot be determined.

Basic Food Groups—In the USDA food intake patterns, the basic food groups are grains; fruits; vegetables; milk, yogurt, and cheese; and meat, poultry, fish, dried peas and beans, eggs, and nuts. In the DASH Eating Plan, nuts, seeds, and dry beans are a separate food group from meat, poultry, fish, and eggs.

Body Mass Index (BMI)—BMI is a practical measure for approximating total body fat and is a measure of weight in relation to height. It is calculated as weight in kilograms divided by the square of the height in meters.

Cardiovascular Disease—Refers to diseases of the heart and diseases of the blood vessel system (arteries, capillaries, veins) within a person's entire body, such as the brain, legs, and lungs.

Cholesterol—A sterol present in all animal tissues. Free cholesterol is a component of cell membranes and serves as a precursor for steroid hormones, including estrogen, testosterone, aldosterone, and bile acids. Humans are able to synthesize sufficient cholesterol to meet biologic requirements, and there is no evidence for a dietary requirement for cholesterol.

- **Dietary cholesterol**—Consumed from foods of animal origin, including meat, fish, poultry, eggs, and dairy products. Plant foods, such as grains, fruits and vegetables, and oils from these sources contain no dietary cholesterol.

- **Serum cholesterol**—Travels in the blood in distinct particles containing both lipids and proteins. Three major classes of lipoproteins are found in the serum of a fasting individual: low-density lipoprotein (LDL), high-density lipoprotein (HDL), and very-low-density lipoprotein (VLDL). Another lipoprotein class, intermediate-density lipoprotein (IDL), resides between VLDL and LDL; in clinical practice, IDL is included in the LDL measurement.

Chronic Diseases—Such as heart disease, cancer, and diabetes—are the leading causes of death and disability in the United States. These diseases account for 7 of every 10 deaths and affect the quality of life of 90 million Americans. Although chronic diseases are among the most common and costly health problems, they are also among the most preventable. Adopting healthy behaviors such as eating nutritious foods, being physically active, and avoiding tobacco use can prevent or control the devastating effects of these diseases.

Coronary Heart Disease—A narrowing of the small blood vessels that supply blood and oxygen to the heart (coronary arteries).

Daily Food Intake Pattern—Identifies the types and amounts of foods that are recommended to be eaten each day and that meet specific nutritional goals. (*Federal Register Notice*, vol. 68, no. 176, p. 53536, Thursday, September 11, 2003.)

Danger Zone—The temperature that allows bacteria to multiply rapidly and produce toxins, between 40°F and 140°F. To keep food out of this danger zone, keep cold food cold and hot food hot. Keep food cold in the refrigerator, in coolers, or on ice in the service line. Keep hot food in the oven, in heated chafing dishes, or in preheated steam tables, warming trays, and/or slow cookers. Never leave perishable foods, such as meat, poultry, eggs, and casseroles, in the danger zone longer than 2 hours or longer than 1 hour in temperatures above 90°F.

Dietary Fiber—Nonstarch polysaccharides and lignin that are not digested by enzymes in the small intestine. Dietary fiber typically refers to nondigestable carbohydrates from plant foods.

Dietary Reference Intakes (DRIs)—A set of nutrient-based reference values that expand upon and replace the former Recommended Dietary Allowances (RDAs) in the United States and the Recommended Nutrient Intakes (RNIs) in Canada. They are actually a set of four reference values: Estimated Average Requirements (EARs), RDAs, AIs, and Tolerable Upper Intake Levels (ULs).

Discretionary Calorie Allowance—The balance of calories remaining in a person's energy allowance after accounting for the number of calories needed to meet recommended nutrient intakes through consumption of foods in low-fat or no-added-sugar forms. The discretionary calorie allowance may be used in selecting forms of foods that are not the most nutrient-dense (e.g., whole milk rather than fat-free milk) or may be additions to foods (e.g., salad dressing, sugar, butter).

Energy Allowance—A person's energy allowance is the calorie intake at which weight maintenance occurs.

Estimated Average Requirements (EARs)—The average daily nutrient intake level estimated to meet the requirement of half the healthy individuals in a particular life stage and gender group.

Estimated Energy Requirement (EER)— Represents the average dietary energy intake that will maintain energy balance in a healthy person of a given gender, age, weight, height, and physical activity level.

FDAMA (Food and Drug Administration Modernization Act)—This act, enacted November 21, 1997, amended the Federal Food, Drug, and Cosmetic Act relating to the regulation of food, drugs, devices, and biological products. With the passage of FDAMA, Congress enhanced the FDA's mission in ways that recognized the agency would be operating in a 21st century characterized by increasing technological, trade, and public health complexities.

FightBAC!—A national public education campaign to promote food safety to consumers and educate them on how to handle and prepare food safely. In this campaign, pathogens are represented by a cartoon-like bacterium character named "BAC."

Food-borne Disease—Caused by consuming contaminated foods or beverages. Many different disease-causing microbes, or pathogens, can contaminate foods, so there are many different food-borne infections. In addition, poisonous chemicals, or other harmful substances, can cause food-borne diseases if they are present in food. The most commonly recognized food-borne infections are those caused by the bacteria *Campylobacter, Salmonella*, and *E. coli* O157:H7, and by a group of viruses called calicivirus, also known as the Norwalk and Norwalk-like viruses.

Heme Iron—One of two forms of iron occurring in foods. Heme iron is bound within the iron-carrying proteins (hemoglobin and myoglobin) found in meat, poultry, and fish. While it contributes a smaller portion of iron to typical American diets than non-heme iron, a larger proportion of heme iron is absorbed.

High Fructose Corn Syrup (HFCS)—A corn sweetener derived from the wet milling of corn. Cornstarch is converted to a syrup that is nearly all dextrose. HFCS is found in numerous foods and beverages on the grocery store shelves.

Hydrogenation—A chemical reaction that adds hydrogen atoms to an unsaturated fat, thus saturating it and making it solid at room temperature.

Leisure-time Physical Activity—Physical activity that is performed during exercise, recreation, or any additional time other than that associated with one's regular job duties, occupation, or transportation.

Listeriosis—A serious infection caused by eating food contaminated with the bacterium *Listeria monocytogenes*, which has recently been recognized as an important public health problem in the United States. The disease affects primarily pregnant women, their fetuses, newborns, and adults with weakened immune systems. Listeria is killed by pasteurization and cooking; however, in certain ready-to-eat foods, such as hot dogs and deli meats, contamination may occur after cooking/manufacture but before packaging. *Listeria monocytogenes* can survive at refrigerated temperatures.

Macronutrient—The dietary macronutrient groups are carbohydrates, proteins, and fats.

Micronutrient—Vitamins and minerals that are required in the human diet in very small amounts.

Moderate Physical Activity—Any activity that burns 3.5 to 7 kcal/minute or the equivalent of 3 to 6 metabolic equivalents (METs), and results in achieving 60% to 73% of peak heart rate. An estimate of a person's peak heart rate can be obtained by subtracting the person's age from 220. Examples of moderate physical activity include walking briskly, mowing the lawn, dancing, swimming, or bicycling on level terrain. A person should feel some exertion but should be able to carry on a conversation comfortably during the activity.

Monounsaturated Fatty Acids (MUFAs)—Monounsaturated fatty acids have one double bond. Plant sources that are rich in MUFAs include vegetable oils (e.g., canola oil, olive oil, high oleic safflower and sunflower oils) that are liquid at room temperature and nuts.

Nutrient-dense Foods—Nutrient-dense foods are those that provide substantial amounts of vitamins and minerals and relatively fewer calories.

Ounce-Equivalent—In the grains food group, the amount of a food counted as equal to a one-ounce slice of bread; in the meat, poultry, fish, dry beans, eggs, and nuts food group, the amount of food counted as equal to one ounce of cooked meat, poultry, or fish. Examples are listed in Appendix C.

Pathogen—Any microorganism that can cause or is capable of causing disease.

Polyunsaturated Fatty Acids (PUFAs)—Polyunsaturated fatty acids have two or more double bonds and may be of two types, based on the position of the first double bond.

- n-6 PUFAs—Linoleic acid, one of the n-6 fatty acids, is required but cannot be synthesized by humans and, therefore, is considered essential in the diet. Primary sources are liquid vegetable oils, including soybean oil, corn oil, and safflower oil.
- n-3 PUFAs—α-linolenic acid is an n-3 fatty acid that is required because it is not synthesized by humans and, therefore, is considered essential in the diet. It is obtained from plant sources, including soybean oil, canola oil, walnuts, and flaxseed. Eicosapentaenoic acid (EPA) and docosahexaenoic acid (DHA) are long-chain n-3 fatty acids contained in fish and shellfish.

Portion Size—The amount of a food consumed in one eating occasion.

Recommended Dietary Allowance (RDA)—The dietary intake level sufficient to meet the nutrient requirement of nearly all (97% to 98%) healthy individuals in a particular life stage gender group.

Resistance Exercise—Anaerobic training, including weight training, weight machine use, and resistance band workouts. Resistance training will increase strength, muscular endurance, and muscle size, while running and jogging will not.

Saturated Fatty Acids—Saturated fatty acids have no double bonds. They primarily come from animal products such as meat and dairy products. In general, animal fats are solid at room temperature.

Sedentary Behaviors—In scientific literature, sedentary is often defined in terms of little or no physical activity during leisure time. A sedentary lifestyle is a lifestyle characterized by little or no physical activity.

Serving Size—A standardized amount of a food, such as a cup or an ounce, used in providing dietary guidance or in making comparisons among similar foods.

Tolerable Upper Intake Level (UL)—The highest average daily nutrient intake level likely to pose no risk of adverse health affects for nearly all individuals in a particular life stage and gender group. As intake increases above the UL, the potential risk of adverse health affects increases.

Trans fatty acids—*Trans* fatty acids, or *trans* fats, are unsaturated fatty acids that contain at least one nonconjugated double bond in the *trans* configuration. Sources of *trans* fatty acids include hydrogenated/partially hydrogenated vegetable oils that are used to make shortening and commercially prepared baked goods, snack foods, fried foods, and margarine. *Trans* fatty acids also are present in foods that come from ruminant animals (e.g., cattle and sheep). Such foods include dairy products, beef, and lamb.

Vegetarian—There are several categories of vegetarians, all of whom avoid meat and/or animal products. The vegan or total vegetarian diet includes only foods from plants: fruits, vegetables, legumes (dried beans and peas), grains, seeds, and nuts. The lacto-vegetarian diet includes plant foods plus cheese and other dairy products. The ovo-lactovegetarian (or lacto-ovovegetarian) diet includes eggs. Semi-vegetarians do not eat red meat but include chicken and fish with plant foods, dairy products, and eggs.

Vigorous Physical Activity—Any activity that burns more than 7 kcal/minute or the equivalent of 6 or more metabolic equivalents (METs), and results in achieving 74% to 88% of peak heart rate. An estimate of a person's peak heart rate can be obtained by subtracting the person's age from 220. Examples of vigorous physical activity include jogging, mowing the lawn with a nonmotorized push mower, chopping wood, participating in high-impact aerobic dancing, swimming continuous laps, or bicycling uphill. Vigorous-intensity physical activity may be intense enough to represent a substantial challenge to an individual and results in a significant increase in heart and breathing rates.

Weight-bearing Exercise—Any activity one performs that works bones and muscles against gravity, including walking, running, hiking, dancing, gymnastics, and soccer.

Whole Grains—Foods made from the entire grain seed, usually called the kernel, which consists of the bran, germ, and endosperm. If the kernel has been cracked, crushed, or flaked, it must retain nearly the same relative proportions of bran, germ, and endosperm as the original grain in order to be called whole grain.*

*AACC Press Release, AACC to Create Consumer-Friendly Whole Grain Definition, March 5, 2004. http://www.aaccnet.org/news/CFWholeGrain.asp from the USDA Dietary Guidelines for Americans 2005. http://www.health.gov/dietaryguidelines/dga2005/document/html/appendixC.htm August 2, 2005.

REFERENCES

American Diabetes Association. (2005). Standards of medical care in diabetes. *Diabetes Care,* (S1), 28, 4–36.

American Psychiatric Association. (2000). *Diagnostic and statistical manual of mental disorders (4th ed.).* Washington, D.C.: American Psychiatric Association.

Finkelstein, E. A., Fiebelkom, I. C., Wang, G. (2003). National medical spending attributable to overweight and obesity: How much, and who's paying? *Health Affairs,* 2003 no. 3, 219–226.

Frantz, M., Bantle, J., Beebe, C., Chiasson, J., Barg, A., Holzmeister, L., Hoogwerf, B., Mayer-Davis, E., Mooradian, A., Purnell, J., Wheeler, M. (2002). Evidence-based nutrition principles and recommendations for the treatment and prevention of diabetes and related complications. *Diabetes Care,* 25, 148–198.

Hockenberry, M. (2005). *Wong's essentials of pediatric nursing* (7th ed). St. Louis: Elsevier Mosby.

Hockenberry, M. (2004). *Wong's clinical manual of pediatric nursing.* St. Louis: Elsevier Mosby.

Stanfield, P. (2003). *Nutrition and diet therapy* (4th ed.). Boston: Jones and Bartlett Publishers.

Useful Web Sites:

http://www.cdc.gov/nccdphp/dnpa/obesity
http://www.cdc.gov/nccdphp/dnpa/bmi
http://www.cdc.gov/alcohol/factsheets/general_information.htm
http://www.health.org
http://www.niaaa.nih.gov
http://www.health.gov/dietaryguidelines/dga2005/document
http://www.healthyplace.com/Communities/Eating_Disorders/index11. asp
http://www.mypyramid.gov
http://www.mypyramid.gov/pyramid/vegetarian.html